MAXIMIZING THIRD-PARTY REIMBURSEMENT IN YOUR MENTAL HEALTH PRACTICE

Richard F. Small, PhD

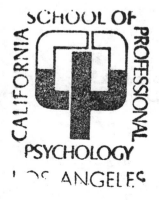

Professional Resource Exchange
Sarasota, Florida

Copyright © 1991 Professional Resource Exchange, Inc.
Professional Resource Exchange, Inc.
635 South Orange Avenue, Suites 4-6
Post Office Box 15560
Sarasota, FL 34277-1560

Printed in the United States of America

Paperbound Edition ISBN: 0-943158-66-4
Library of Congress Catalog Card Number: 91-52551

The copy editor for this book was Patricia Hammond, the proofreader was Jack Winner, the managing editor was Debbie Fink, the graphics coordinator was Laurie Girsch, and the cover designer was Bill Tabler.

ACKNOWLEDGEMENTS

I would like to thank the many people who provided articles, information, and advice of all kinds. I would particularly like to recognize Samuel Knapp, EdD, for a wealth of information as well as for a "fine-tooth" review of my manuscript. My heart-felt thanks go to my wife, Mindy Sue Small, for typing, editing, and furnishing me with many ideas. Finally, I appreciate the support of my children, Dylan and Liz, for their encouragement and patience during a project that occupied more of my time than any of us anticipated.

TABLE OF CONTENTS

MAXIMIZING
THIRD-PARTY
REIMBURSEMENT
IN YOUR
MENTAL HEALTH PRACTICE

CHAPTER 1
INTRODUCTION

I entered independent practice in 1979, shortly after the passage of Act 16 of 1978, Pennsylvania's "Freedom of Choice" law for psychologists. It quickly became apparent that understanding health insurance and third-party reimbursement would be an important key to a successful psychological practice. Because psychotherapy is "labor-intensive" and therefore expensive, honest discussion of finances and insurance would be important in establishing a therapeutic relationship. If not addressed, these issues could otherwise become an unspoken barrier to effective psychotherapy. My realization of the importance of keeping abreast of continually changing insurance issues led to my becoming Chair of the Insurance Committee of the Pennsylvania Psychological Association, presentation of numerous workshops and articles, and, finally, this book.

Unfortunately, many mental health professionals are disinclined to become informed about a subject so essential to their livelihood. Many practitioners have closed their eyes, claiming "I am not a businessperson," while complaining about rent, expenses, lack of referrals, and inadequate appreciation (i.e., monetary compensation) for the difficult job of being a therapist. Others say that they would like to understand insurance and reimbursement better but do not know where to look. At workshops, participants frequently comment that colleagues seem unwilling to honestly share practical details relating to their practices. In recent years, journal articles and books have appeared that address global reimbursement issues, but few deal with the "nuts and bolts" of how patients and therapists get paid by third parties.

My goal is to present a readable, practical guide to third-party reimbursement. Explanations of insurance terms and concepts are provided to give practitioners a perspective and database so that they can evaluate unique situations that will affect their practices. Ethical issues and dilemmas are discussed. Because appropriate solutions to some ethical problems are not nearly as obvious as some writers suggest, I offer a range of solutions formulated by various practitioners and commentators. Along with the more formal explanations of insurance regulations and procedures, I have included many suggestions from my colleagues and my own experiences.

Changes in health care reimbursement occur so rapidly that my words are becoming outdated even as they are being written. To help alleviate this problem, I have attempted to present the broad picture as well as specifics, so that this book will be useful for quite a few years. Although particulars may change greatly, many of the general ideas will remain the same. It is vital for practitioners to stay abreast of third-party reimbursement developments through their state association newsletters, national association newspapers (e.g., the *American Psychological Association Monitor, Psychiatric News, NASW NEWS, Marriage and Family Therapist*), periodicals such as *Psychotherapy Finances*, and bulletins provided by the insurance carriers.

Medicare, CHAMPUS, and other federal programs vary little from state to state. On the other hand, Blue Cross/Blue Shield and Medical Assistance (Medicaid) may be very different among states. Private insurance plans vary greatly among employers. Practitioners who want to stay knowledgeable about their patients' insurance reimbursement must understand the insurance plans offered by major local employers. It is also important to realize that reimbursement policies often change from year to year, even if an individual is employed by the same company.

A basic theme underlying this book is that it is in the interest of all mental health practitioners, whether or not they choose to become directly involved in their patients' insurance claims, to understand third-party reimbursement issues. Decisions about how much a therapist will help patients obtain reimbursement affect the image and character of the practice. These choices are integrated with such decisions as whether the therapist usually requires payment at each session or is willing to bill patients, and the amount of help the office will provide. The therapist's involvement or noninvolvement in insurance reimbursement has a major impact on the therapeutic relationship. Some practitioners may find that active involvement in reimbursement issues interferes with psychotherapeutic work. Others see such help as enhancing the patient's view of the therapist as "caring." Providing assistance with insurance reimbursement, accepting assignment, or being a participating provider may increase referrals and strengthen a practice. On the other hand, these actions create paperwork, take time, and may ultimately involve lower fees per patient.

In summary, I believe that all practitioners need a solid understanding of insurance and reimbursement issues. Only then can they make choices as to how they will handle their practices in the informed context of all the therapeutic, financial, and practice-building nuances.

PRACTITIONER ATTITUDES

Many practitioners see reimbursement issues as unprofessional and mercenary, refusing to be involved in, or even informed about them. Yet most of these same therapists would like both to serve their clients in the best possible manner and enjoy the financial benefits of their hard work. In therapy, these clinicians readily concur that their patients' monetary worries, needs, and goals are highly significant, appropriate, and worthy concerns. Yet they may perceive their own thoughts about being paid for therapeutic services as "impure." Because they see themselves as *helpers* rather than *businesspeople*, they construe examining issues such as fees and nonpayment as distasteful.

I believe these therapists are ignoring important realities of independent practice. I have compared my fees to the actual cost of services in mental health centers, which are often provided by less credentialed and less experienced individuals, with a high rate of turnover. The cost per hour for my clinical time is often similar, and sometimes less expensive, than clinic charges. I can provide quality, cost-effective, caring treatment and also earn a reasonably good living. Only by looking at financial issues, including my patients' opportunities for reimbursement, can I fulfill my potential as a private therapist.

Lane and Hull (1990) claim that the "manner in which the fee is handled or not handled by the therapist may be expected to have pervasive and profound effects on therapy" (p. 260). They cite various authorities who agree that awareness of the therapeutic impact of fees and reimbursement is necessary. If the therapist ignores these issues, it is likely to have a deleterious effect upon the therapy.

Other common practitioner attitudes are either "I can't be bothered" or "it's your [the patient's] problem." Both attitudes are short-sighted. The short-term inconvenience of attending to reimbursement issues leads to long-term gains of more referrals, a busier practice, patients who can continue in treatment, and a more positive relationship between the therapist and client.

Some therapists are well educated about insurance reimbursement, have carefully considered the pros and cons, and then elect noninvolvement. A number of my colleagues do no billing, ask for full payment at each session, and do not complete insurance forms. They will provide superbills, or statements with diagnoses, so that patients can obtain reimbursement on their own. These therapists have decided that the paperwork and risk of noncollection outweigh the advantages of more active involvement. In fact, the North Carolina Psychological Association Insurance Committee (1989) seems to recommend this method. Langs (1976) goes even further by not even providing statements with diagnoses because he feels this practice would interfere with the "therapeutic frame."

Kovacs (1988) opposes tying psychologists' futures to third party payers. He found that between 1958 and 1978, the proportion of his patients' fees coming from insurance reimbursement rose from 0% to 65%, but declined to 20% of his gross practice revenues by 1988. Kovacs views most managed-care proposals as ways to contain costs rather than to increase or improve services, since they encourage participation by salaried providers with limited training. He advocates establishing psychology as a *human service* fee-for-service profession similar to attorneys, accountants, architects, and estate planners, rather than as a *health care* profession. Human service professions are seen as offering services that clients perceive as "important, significant, even vital -- and well worth paying for" (pp. 25-26). Currently, patients often see payment for psychotherapy, like most other health services, as the responsibility of the therapist and the insurance company. Kovacs' ideas, while directed particularly to psychologists, are applicable to other mental health professionals. Even psychiatrists, who fit best into a health delivery model, are often being inadequately reimbursed for psychotherapy.

At this time, I have chosen to be very involved in insurance reimbursement. I see my practice as one that provides the best possible service to my clients. This includes not only my best therapy and clinical assessment but also an office that conveys concern about patients' pleasantness, convenience, and anything else that will enhance the therapeutic relationship.

When prospective patients call, I review the clinical information, assess whether an initial interview is appropriate, and explain my fee. I ask whether they have health insurance and give them information about probable coverage. I do not guarantee the accuracy of the information (insurance policies can change so quickly) and suggest that they check with their employer or insurer as to the specifics of their plan. I also state that payment is ultimately the patient's responsibility. Nevertheless, my office offers to be of maximum help in obtaining reimbursement. Specifics of how we handle different types of insurance will be discussed later in the book. I view our active, involved approach as a part of a professional, highly personalized practice.

PATIENT ATTITUDES

Before closing this chapter, it is important to look at common attitudes that patients have about fees and reimbursement. Since World War II, employed individuals increasingly have expected insurance to cover most of their health care costs. In the past 20 years, coverage for dental and optical services has been included more and more in the health care package. Employers and insurance companies often tout their policies as high quality and "the best there is." Unfortunately, mental health coverage often gets short shrift, even in otherwise good health care policies.

Patients seeking mental health services often feel entitled to full coverage. They may be angry at the therapist if there are out-of-pocket costs. When prospective patients call and we discuss insurance, they frequently say "Don't worry, we have the best coverage." I am often familiar with their plans, which may be extremely limited for psychological services, and will inform them of the approximate coverage. Although I may repeat this information, they often do not "hear" and after the treatment has begun are shocked and angry that they must pay.

Like the therapist who shrugs and says to the patient "It's your problem," many patients will say to the therapist "It's your problem." Despite telephone preparation, they arrive at my office with only an insurance form, clearly indicating that they expect to bear no personal financial responsibility. Even more irritating are the patients who do not even bring an insurance form, tell me that I can call their employer or insurance company for forms and information, and totally absent themselves from any involvement or obligation.

Another delicate situation, for those therapists seeing children, involves divorce. Frequently the custodial parent says that the former spouse, who may or may not be willing to be a part of the therapy, is responsible for payment. We indicate a willingness to work with the ex-spouse and his or her insurance company, but make it clear that the parent bringing the child is ultimately responsible for payment. Mistakes made early in my practice have made me aware of how the therapist's fee can easily become one more part of the vicious battle between divorcing or divorced spouses.

DISCLAIMER

All attempts have been made to provide information that is accurate at the time this book was written. However, some of the specific information provided is likely to become out-of-date because federal and state regulations are constantly changing and because the health care reimbursement industry is also changing very rapidly.

Furthermore, although legal issues may be discussed, nothing in this book should be construed as legal advice. All opinions, unless otherwise stated, are those of the author. Readers with questions about specific coverage, ethics, or legal issues in a particular case are advised to consult the specific employer, insurance company, state or federal agency, professional organization, or the therapist's personal attorney.

CHAPTER 2
BASIC CONCEPTS

Before getting into the "nuts and bolts" of filing forms, it is necessary to understand basic insurance terms. Like other specialized fields, the insurance industry has a unique jargon, known only to insiders, and has unique rules and procedures. This chapter explains these basic ideas and terms.

THIRD-PARTY REIMBURSEMENT AND INSURANCE

Although both practitioners and patients use the words "insurance" and "third party" many times a day, few people understand what these terms actually mean. A "third party" is any person or entity that pays for services on behalf of a patient (Stromberg et al., 1988). A third party may be an employer, insurance company, government agency, or even a parent or friend. Payment may be partial or for the entire service. Traditionally, although third parties asked for confirmation that services had been performed and for minimal additional information such as a diagnosis, they did not actively involve themselves in the treatment process. With managed care, third parties may ask for a great deal more information and are becoming increasingly involved in treatment decisions.

It is important to distinguish the therapist-patient contract from the compact between a patient and the insurance company or other third-party provider. Generally, the therapist agrees to perform services and the patient agrees to pay for them. The patient's contract with the insurance company is independent of the therapist-patient agreement, and the therapist's payment should not be contingent upon the patient's receipt of reimbursement. If the therapist has contracted with a third-party reimburser (e.g., by becoming a "participating provider"), the patient is obligated to pay only co-payments or deductibles.

Until recently *indemnity insurance* was the predominant model of third-party health care reimbursement, but it now competes with other forms. Indemnity insurance is usually referred to simply as *insurance*, to be distinguished from other concepts such as Health Maintenance Organizations. Under an indemnity insurance plan, an individual or employer pays a specific premium to cover unanticipated costs. We insure our cars, our houses, and even our lives. Insurance exists not because we *expect* accidents, fires, damage, or death, but because these things *could* happen, and their financial impact would be very adverse. Health insurance should be a premium paid to cover *unanticipated* medical expenses. Certain provisions, such as routine mammograms and dental check-ups, are not truly "insurance," but rather are benefits that insurance companies have added to make their policies more attractive. These added benefits result in increased premiums.

Mental health practitioners, as well as the public at large, often fail to understand insurance. Insurance companies are usually private enterprises designed to make a profit by providing a legitimate service. Through *financial risk sharing* the cost of protecting against major, unanticipated expenses becomes more affordable because one person's risk is shared among many others over time. This reduces the vulnerability of an individual (or even small group) to infrequent, large financial liabilities in exchange for a much smaller payment (Baughman, 1989). The "risk pool" must be large enough so that an individual catastrophe will have little effect on premium rates.

As psychotherapists, we often decry the absence of unlimited mental health coverage. As consumers, we complain about our own dramatically rising health insurance premiums, but at the same time we do not want our coverage cut back. Ironically, group plans for mental health professionals often severely restrict their coverage of mental health services. Because mental health professionals tend to be more convinced of the usefulness of psychotherapy, their utilization of mental health services is often greater. Insurance companies would lose money if they provided unlimited mental health benefits to mental health groups, unless they charged very high premiums.

It is most important to insure oneself against catastrophic loss. Although an individual of some means might reasonably consider risking the loss of a $3,000 car by not having collision insurance, it would be folly to forego liability insurance, because one might successfully be sued for a million dollars. Similarly, a health insurance policy with a low premium which does not reimburse the first $500, or even $5,000, of health costs, might be advantageous for many individuals. On the other hand, enrolling in a health plan with no deductible, but a $10,000 maximum payment, would probably be unwise, because one catastrophic illness could cost $100,000 or more and wipe out most families' total assets.

Unfortunately, most mental health coverage violates basic insurance logic. Frequently, there are low per-session payments, limits on the number of sessions, and low yearly and lifetime maximums. Individuals who need a minimal or moderate amount of mental health care may find themselves adequately covered. Yet people who need more extensive treatment often have inadequate coverage and face the choice of foregoing necessary care or facing financial devastation.

TYPES OF INSURANCE

Most of this book concerns itself with *health insurance*. Whether provided through the government, an employer, or an individual contract between subscriber and insurance company, health insurance provides reimbursement for certain expenses incurred in treatment (including cure and/or rehabilitation) of illness. "Mental illness" may be included, as specifically defined by the insurance company. For instance, certain policies will not cover "personality disorders." Virtually all policies require services to be "medically necessary and appropriate care" and allow the insurance company or third-party administrator to make that determination.

Other types of insurance may include mental health services. Employers are required to purchase *workers' compensation* policies and reimburse employees for costs of injuries incurred in the course of their employment. Mental health coverage may be available for anxiety or depression associated with a physical work-related injury, or for purely psychological symptoms resulting from a work situation. For example, a bank teller might require treatment for severe anxiety following an armed bank robbery, even though there was no physical injury. The eligibility of various mental health professionals for reimbursement under workers' compensation policies varies, depending on the insurance company and state law.

Most *automobile* policies include some coverage for medical treatment. These may include the psychological effects of automobile accidents. Mental health services may also be covered under *homeowner's* and various *corporate liability* policies, including product liability.

Professional liability (malpractice) insurance, a subject of interest to all mental health practitioners, does not fall into the same category as those mentioned previously. These policies would not be a potential source of reimbursement for a mental health practitioner (except as a patient or an expert witness). This insurance protects practitioners from damages in justified or unjustified malpractice lawsuits.

Major medical plans were designed as "umbrella" coverage to pay for large expenses that other health insurance plans do not cover. For example, Blue Cross pays most hospital costs, while Blue Shield pays doctors' fees associated with hospitalization. Major medical was designed as a program with a low premium to cover the "unlikely" occurrence of catastrophic illnesses that exceeded the coverage of Blue Cross and Blue Shield. As people wanted more health coverage, benefits were added to Blue Cross, Blue Shield, and major medical. Therefore, "regular" health insurance often covers most inpatient mental health costs, while outpatient care often falls under the major medical policy.

Most insurance has traditionally followed a *fee-for-service* model, in which practitioners charge the patient (or insurance company) for each separate service delivered. Some newer health coverage programs attempt to reduce costs by utilizing different reimbursement formulas. For example, the Diagnosis Related Group (DRG) system involves paying per illness and thereby discourages unnecessary services. Health Maintenance Organizations (HMOs) pay a flat fee for each enrollee regardless of how many services each individual requires.

DEDUCTIBLES, CO-PAYMENTS, MAXIMUMS, AND LIMITS

Most insurance plans include a yearly *deductible*, an amount which must be paid by the patient before any insurance benefits will start. The *benefit period*, usually 1 year, does not always coincide with a calendar year. The deductible, which usually ranges from $50 to $1,000, is likely to apply to all health-related expenses but occasionally counts only against mental health expenses. Deductibles may apply to individual family members or to the family as a whole. For example, a policy may have a $200 deductible for each family member, but when total family expenses exceed $500, the deductible may be met, regardless of whether each family member has reached $200.

Most insurance policies include a *co-payment* for mental health services. The patient is responsible for this portion of the therapist's fee. The co-payment may be a set dollar amount but is more likely to be a percentage of the fee, usually from 20% to 80%. Co-payments often apply only to outpatient services, or may be lower for inpatients.

Some policies establish *stop-loss limits*. When the stop-loss limit is reached (usually when allowed charges exceed $1,000 to $5,000), the insurance reimbursement becomes 100%, subject to yearly and lifetime maximums. Mental health services are often exempted from the stop-loss limits.

Insurance companies impose many *maximums* and *limits* on mental health coverage. There may be a lifetime maximum, which usually includes inpatient and outpatient services (often $25,000 or less); a yearly maximum, which may separate inpatient and outpatient services and can be as low as $500; and/or a per-session maximum. For example, a company might have 50% payment with a $40 maximum charge. If the therapist's fee is $100, the insurance would pay only $20 (i.e., 50% of $40). Thus, what appears to be 50% coverage in the employee's insurance manual, is - in reality - only 20% coverage.

ASSIGNMENT AND PARTICIPATING PROVIDERS

Assignment is a legal "transfer to another person of part or all of one's rights or obligations under a contract, transaction or law" (Stromberg et al., 1988, p. 199). Under most private plans, assignment is on a claim-by-claim basis and does not obligate practitioners to limit their fees. If a patient assigns insurance payments to the provider, the third party will mail payment directly to the practitioner. In most private insurance plans this involves no obligation on the provider's part. In order to receive assignment for Medicare, Blue Shield, and many managed-care programs, one must agree to accept the insurance carrier's determination of a maximum fee. For example, if a therapist with a usual charge of $100 agrees to participate in a plan with a 50% co-payment and maximum fee of $80, the insurance company will pay the provider $40, and it is the provider's responsibility to collect the other $40 from the patient. The provider cannot collect more. If it is a private plan and the therapist has not agreed to be a participating provider, and the patient has allowed assignment, the therapist would receive a check for $40 and would be entitled to collect $60 from the patient.

USUAL, CUSTOMARY, AND
REASONABLE (UCR) PLAN

Blue Shield, Medicare, and many private insurance plans have traditionally operated under a *usual, customary, and reasonable (UCR)* plan. Insurance companies will often establish an *Individual Provider Profile* for each practitioner or group. This profile is a compilation of past charges by a practitioner. As charges increase, the profile also increases, although there is usually a lag of a year or more. The *usual* fee is that provider's most frequent charge for the procedure performed.

The *customary* charge is based upon the insurance company's compilation of the fees of providers with similar training in a given geographic area for a specific procedure. Insurers calculate the charges of similar providers in a region and pay no more than the 70th to 90th percentile. Thus, if 90% of social workers in a given area charge $90 or less, a social worker charging $125 as a usual fee would be reimbursed no more than $90 under a UCR plan using the 90th percentile. Since 1984, most insurance plans, including many Blue Cross/Blue Shield plans and Medicare, have artificially limited the rate of increase in customary fees.

The *reasonable* fee is determined by the insurance company and applies to unusual circumstances. For example, although a policy might limit reimbursement to one hour-long session per day, if it could be demonstrated that an individual had a severe suicidal or homicidal crisis requiring a 2-hour intervention, the insurance company might consider accepting a charge higher than the usual 1-hour UCR to be *reasonable*. It is my experience that getting insurance companies to allow more than the usual or customary charge is extremely rare and requires more time than the service itself might have taken.

UCR fees are "provider driven"; that is, they increase only as providers increase their charges. UCRs also tend to lag behind providers' actual fees by a year or more, which creates an incentive for practitioners to raise fees in anticipation of a need for higher fees. Therefore, UCRs are often seen as contributing to higher costs and seem to be disappearing as a system for establishing health care reimbursement rates.

FREEDOM OF CHOICE, SELF-INSURANCE, AND ERISA

Before 1973, most insurance policies limited mental health benefits to services provided by physicians. In 1973 New Jersey passed the first *Freedom of Choice Law*, requiring insurance companies that reimburse physicians for mental health services to also reimburse psychologists for these same services. Since that time, more than 40 states, representing more than 85% of the American population, have enacted similar legislation. Freedom of Choice for social workers has become law in 15 states. Inclusion of counselors as well as marriage and family therapists has been passed by several state legislatures and introduced in many others ("Practice Issues: Social Workers," 1987; Stromberg et al., 1988; Whiting, 1989).

Self-insured companies underwrite and provide insurance benefits for their employees. The company often sets up an insurance trust to which it contributes. Sometimes these insurance trusts are "insured" in turn by other companies. This limit on self-insured losses makes their legal status somewhat problematic.

A threat to Freedom of Choice comes from the Employees Retirement Income Security Act (ERISA). This law protects pension funds by "preempting" or nullifying state insurance codes as they apply to "self-insured" employee benefit plans. It excludes such plans from the definition of insurance. Many corporations have set up plans of "self-insurance" and have excluded psychologists, social workers, and other providers, despite Freedom of Choice laws in those states. (These issues will be explored in-depth in Chapter 5.)

MANAGED CARE

Managed care is a term that emerged in the late 1980s but is usually left undefined. Small (1989) says that "managed care is not a legal term, but seems to include any plan that attempts to control the cost of health care by setting limits on reimbursement" (p. 12). True *insurance* plans may control costs through utilization review, precertification, and other means. Health maintenance organizations (HMOs), preferred provider organizations (PPOs), independent practice associations (IPAs), and an alphabet soup of other organizations have been devised to attempt to contain costs.

Although they have only become widespread in recent years, *HMOs* have a long history. HMOs pay flat fees *(capitation)* to providers for all health care services, regardless of utilization. In principle, this encourages providers to keep patients healthy at the lowest cost, and avoid unnecessary procedures. Unfortunately, it also risks encouraging inadequate care. Specialty services, including mental health, may be provided by HMO providers on a capitation or a fee-for-service basis, or may be referred to others.

A *PPO* controls costs by providing services at a discount. The providers agree to charge less for their services in exchange for more referrals. PPO providers may be restricted to particular groups, such as the medical staff members of a particular hospital, participating members of the National Register of Health Service Providers in Psychology, or other organizations.

Despite the proliferation of letters and acronyms, most managed-care organizations seem to be hybrids of HMOs, PPOs, and other plans. They are evolving as need, demand, and satisfaction change. One might now divide them into those which employ full-time, salaried therapists and those which contract with independent practitioners. The common element for the latter is that the therapist will usually accept a lesser fee in exchange for referrals and guaranteed payment. These programs will be discussed in detail in Chapter 8.

Utilization Review (UR) is an essential component of managed care. Services are subject to approval by the third party, through requiring precertification and/or approval to continue services. Separate UR companies sometimes contract to managed-care organizations and may be referred to as "fourth parties."

EMPLOYEE ASSISTANCE PLANS

Although not insurance, the *Employee Assistance Plan (EAP)* is a benefit that most large corporations have instituted in the last few years, particularly in response to the impact of drug and alcohol abuse. EAPs vary widely in format but typically provide various services including some counseling (often a limit of three to eight sessions) and referrals to private practitioners. EAPs can sometimes supplement mental health insurance coverage. It is likely that EAP and insurance coverage will blend even more in the future.

OTHER INSURANCE TERMS

Diagnosis Related Groups (DRGs) were instituted by Medicare and quickly adopted by other carriers to control hospital costs. Hospitals are paid set amounts for a particular illness or procedure, regardless of the actual length of stay for a particular patient.

Coordination of benefits applies when the patient has multiple insurance contracts. If an individual is covered under his or her own policy as well as the spouse's, and each pays 25%, that individual can usually collect from both carriers. If each carrier pays 80%, the patient is not entitled to 160% of the cost. The *primary carrier* (usually defined by law) pays its agreed percentage (e.g., 80%), and the *secondary carrier* covers part or all of the remaining fee. Patients will be expected to cover whatever costs remain. Medicare is secondary to private carriers. Health insurance is usually secondary to automobile or workers' compensation.

A new twist, which will be increasingly seen, is called a *carve-out* or *maintenance of benefits* approach (Case, 1990). With the traditional coordination of benefits rules, if each carrier covers 50%, the total reimbursement would be 100%. In this situation, the secondary payer makes up the difference between what the primary plan paid and what the secondary carrier would have paid if there were no other insurance. Under the carve-out provisions, the primary insurer would pay the 50% and the secondary insurer would pay nothing.

If an insurance company mistakenly pays a therapist or patient for a service not covered, it is likely to demand repayment. It can deduct the amount from future payments, or even sue the therapist or patient for recovery of these payments.

A carrier will often contract with a group to administer its insurance program and act as an *intermediary*. For example, as of 1990, Blue Cross/Blue Shield of South Carolina was the CHAMPUS intermediary for much of the East Coast. When a carrier acts as an intermediary, it follows the rules and regulations of the host organization rather than those typical of its own policies.

Confusion arises when insurance companies act as intermediaries for self-insured plans. Individuals may mistakenly assume Freedom of Choice coverage when the insurance company is administering rather than insuring.

Most insurance companies limit treatment for *preexisting conditions* to protect themselves from individuals who may contract a serious illness and then obtain insurance. Frequently preexisting mental illnesses are not covered for 1 year. It has been my experience, however, that companies frequently do not enforce their limits on preexisting conditions for mental health services.

Other *exclusions* may include such things as treatment of obesity, "experimental procedures," biofeedback, or hypnosis.

CHAPTER 3
FILING A
HEALTH INSURANCE CLAIM

Figure 1 (p. 16) shows a typical insurance form. Although many companies supply their own, most will accept generic "universal forms" similar to the one shown. The following discussion explains each aspect of completing an insurance form and highlights some major issues.

SECTIONS OF THE FORM

PATIENT AND INSURED INFORMATION (SECTION A)

Much of the *patient and insured information* is obvious, but it is important that it be as accurate and complete as possible. Incomplete information can lead to processing delays, sometimes of many months. Likewise, although the specific designated insurance program (Medicare, Blue Shield, etc.) is usually obvious, when an organization such as Blue Shield administers another program (such as Medicare), the latter is the proper one to mark.

Figure 1 shows some of the complications that may arise in filing an insurance form. In this case the patient, Jason Popp, lives with his remarried mother, Pamela Ironwood, in Iowa. The insured for this policy is his father, James Popp, who lives in Rhode Island.

Although it is common for an insured (or *beneficiary*) to have a different last name than the patient, this seems to cause confusion for many insurance companies. When Pamela Ironwood files a claim for her son, Jason Popp, reimbursement is likely to be listed for services provided to Jason Ironwood. Although Ms. Ironwood may have paid for the service herself, her ex-husband will probably receive the reimbursement check because he is the insured.

RELATIONSHIP TO INSURED (SECTION B)

Insurance policies may also cover stepchildren. The psychotherapy provided by Dr. Charleston may be covered under either the father's, mother's, or stepfather's insur-

HEALTH INSURANCE CLAIM FORM FORM APPROVED OMB NO. 0938-0008

READ INSTRUCTIONS BEFORE COMPLETING OR SIGNING THIS FORM (CHECK APPLICABLE PROGRAM BLOCK BELOW)

☐ MEDICARE (MEDICARE NO.)	☐ MEDICAID (MEDICAID NO.)	☐ CHAMPUS (SPONSOR'S SSN)	☐ CHAMPVA (VA FILE NO.)	☐ FECA BLACK LUNG (SSN)	☒ OTHER (CERTIFICATE SSN)

PATIENT AND INSURED (SUBSCRIBER) INFORMATION

(A)

1. PATIENT'S NAME (LAST NAME, FIRST NAME, MIDDLE INITIAL)
Popp, Jason

2. PATIENT'S DATE OF BIRTH
4 | 24 | 75

3. INSURED'S NAME (LAST NAME, FIRST NAME, MIDDLE INITIAL)
Popp, James

4. PATIENT'S ADDRESS (STREET, CITY, STATE, ZIP CODE)
1214 Cardinal Street
Delaire, IA 52000

TELEPHONE NO. (712) 775-1132

5. PATIENT'S SEX
MALE ☒   FEMALE ☐

6. INSURED'S ID NO. (FOR PROGRAM CHECKED ABOVE, INCLUDE ALL LETTERS)
1944/031850-MSU

(B) 7. PATIENT'S RELATIONSHIP TO INSURED
SELF ☐ SPOUSE ☐ CHILD ☒ OTHER ☐

8. INSURED'S GROUP NO. (OR GROUP NAME OR FECA CLAIM NO.)
121403180319 0424
☒ INSURED IS EMPLOYED AND COVERED BY EMPLOYER HEALTH PLAN

9. OTHER HEALTH INSURANCE COVERAGE (ENTER NAME OF POLICYHOLDER AND PLAN NAME AND ADDRESS AND POLICY OR MEDICAL ASSISTANCE NUMBER)
Pamela Ironwood
No Benefit Insurance Co.
Hartford, CT 06000
#123456789

(C) 10. WAS CONDITION RELATED TO
A. PATIENT'S EMPLOYMENT
YES ☐   NO ☒

B. ACCIDENT
AUTO ☐   OTHER ☐

11. INSURED'S ADDRESS (STREET, CITY, STATE, ZIP CODE)
70 Claverack Avenue
Meadowlane, RI 02000
TELEPHONE NO. (401) 828-2360

11A. CHAMPUS SPONSOR'S
STATUS | ☐ ACTIVE DUTY ☐ DECEASED ☐ RETIRED | BRANCH OF SERVICE

(D) 12. PATIENT'S OR AUTHORIZED PERSON'S SIGNATURE (READ BACK BEFORE SIGNING) I AUTHORIZE THE RELEASE OF ANY MEDICAL INFORMATION NECESSARY TO PROCESS THIS CLAIM. I ALSO REQUEST PAYMENT OF GOVERNMENT BENEFITS EITHER TO MYSELF OR TO THE PARTY WHO ACCEPTS ASSIGNMENT BELOW.
SIGNED Pamela Ironwood   DATE 3/19/91

(E) 13. I AUTHORIZE PAYMENT OF MEDICAL BENEFITS TO UNDERSIGNED PHYSICIAN OR SUPPLIER FOR SERVICE DESCRIBED BELOW.
SIGNED (INSURED OR AUTHORIZED PERSON) James Popp

PHYSICIAN OR SUPPLIER INFORMATION

(F) 14. DATE OF: ILLNESS (FIRST SYMPTOM) OR INJURY (ACCIDENT) OR PREGNANCY (LMP)

15. DATE FIRST CONSULTED YOU FOR THIS CONDITION 3/1/91

16. IF PATIENT HAS HAD SAME OR SIMILAR ILLNESS OR INJURY, GIVE DATES

16A. IF EMERGENCY CHECK HERE

(G) 17. DATE PATIENT ABLE TO RETURN TO WORK

18. DATES OF TOTAL DISABILITY
FROM   THROUGH

DATES OF PARTIAL DISABILITY
FROM   THROUGH

(H) 19. NAME OF REFERRING PHYSICIAN OR OTHER SOURCE (E.G., PUBLIC HEALTH AGENCY)
Cosette Fantine, MD

(I) 20. FOR SERVICES RELATED TO HOSPITALIZATION GIVE HOSPITALIZATION DATES
ADMITTED 3/1/91   DISCHARGED 3/4/91

(J) 21. NAME AND ADDRESS OF FACILITY WHERE SERVICES RENDERED (IF OTHER THAN OFFICE)
Delaire General Hospital, 51 Fifth Ave., Delaire, IA

22. WAS LABORATORY WORK PERFORMED OUTSIDE YOUR OFFICE?
YES ☐   NO ☒   CHARGES

(K) 23A. DIAGNOSIS OR NATURE OF ILLNESS OR INJURY; RELATE DIAGNOSIS TO PROCEDURE IN COL. D BY REFERENCE NOS. 1, 2, 3, ETC. OR DX CODE

1. 300.40 (DSM-III-R) - Dysthymia
2.
3.
4.

23B.
EPSDT   YES ☐   NO ☐
FAMILY PLANNING   YES ☐   NO ☐
PRIOR AUTHORIZATION NO.

(L)

24. A. DATE OF SERVICE FROM – TO	B.* PLACE OF SERVICE	C. PROCEDURE CODE (IDENTIFY) / FULLY DESCRIBE PROCEDURES, MEDICAL SERVICES OR SUPPLIES FURNISHED FOR EACH DATE GIVEN (EXPLAIN UNUSUAL SERVICES OR CIRCUMSTANCES)	D. DIAGNOSIS CODE	E. CHARGES	F. DAYS OR UNITS	G.* T.O.S.	H. LEAVE BLANK
3/1/91	I	-99 90620 75-WD Comprehensive Psychological Consultation 2 hr.	1	200 00			
3/8/91	O	90844 Psychotherapy - Full	1	100 00			
3/15/91	O	90844 Psychotherapy - Full	1	100 00			
3/22/91	O	90844 Psychotherapy - Full	1	100 00			

(M) 25. SIGNATURE OF PHYSICIAN OR SUPPLIER (INCLUDING DEGREE(S) OR CREDENTIALS) (I CERTIFY THAT THE STATEMENTS ON THE REVERSE APPLY TO THIS BILL AND ARE MADE A PART THEREOF.)
Steven J. Charleston PhD
DATE 3/25/91

26. ACCEPT ASSIGNMENT (GOVERNMENT CLAIMS ONLY) (SEE BACK)
YES ☐   NO ☐

27. TOTAL CHARGE
500 00

28. AMOUNT PAID
—

29. BALANCE DUE
500.00

30. YOUR SOCIAL SECURITY NO.
001-10-0001

31. PHYSICIAN'S, SUPPLIER'S, AND/OR GROUP NAME, ADDRESS, ZIP CODE AND TELEPHONE NO.
Stephen J. Charleston, PhD
26 Dartmouth Street
Adamsville, IA 52740
(712) 723-6036
Tax #23-000000
ID NO. IOWA LICENSE # 7776868 PS

32. YOUR PATIENT'S ACCOUNT NO.
171612

33. YOUR EMPLOYER ID NO.
23-000000

*PLACE OF SERVICE AND TYPE OF SERVICE (T.O.S.) CODES ON BACK
REMARKS:

APPROVED BY AMA COUNCIL ON MEDICAL SERVICE 6/83

FORM HCFA-1500 (1-84) FORM OWCP-1500
FORM CHAMPUS-501 (1-84) FORM RRB-1500
APPROVED BY THE HEALTH CARE FINANCING ADMINISTRATION & CHAMPUS

Note. Reprinted with permission of Colwell Systems, Inc., P.O. Box 4024, Champaign, Illinois 61824-4024.

Figure 1. Health Insurance Claim Form.

ance policy. It is often advisable to file with all three companies. Although therapists should never intentionally attempt to obtain reimbursement when a patient is not entitled to such reimbursement, it is not the responsibility of the therapist or patient to determine which policy should take responsibility for primary coverage of the psychotherapy.

It is also unclear, in the case of a stepchild, whether one should check "child" or "other" on the form. In my experience, if the insured is a stepparent of the patient, he or she often checks "child." I do not know of any instances where this has been challenged by any insurance company.

EMPLOYMENT OR ACCIDENT RELATED (SECTION C)

It is important to indicate whether the condition is related to employment or to an accident. Workers' compensation, auto, and other accident policies will generally pay benefits, often at 100%, as primary payer. Thus, if an individual has an automobile policy with $100,000 of medical benefits, the automobile insurer is responsible for physical and mental injury until those costs reach $100,000. At that point, coverage reverts to the medical plan. As a secondary payer, a health insurer will want proof that there is no other coverage before paying these claims.

RELEASE OF INFORMATION (SECTION D)

Box 12 authorizes the practitioner to release any medical information needed to process the claim. Without this signature the therapist does not have explicit permission to provide any information to the insurance company.

The authorization signature should be that of the patient (or guardian), regardless of who is insured. If the husband is the patient and covered under his wife's policy, the husband must give permission for information about him, as a patient, to be released.

Insurance companies may request treatment summaries before processing claims. Occasionally, they will ask for all records. If asked for unreasonable information, it is best to consult with the patient and perhaps an attorney before complying. Progress notes may be irrelevant to the insurer and potentially embarrassing or damaging to the patient.

If especially extensive or time-consuming information is requested, it is not unreasonable for a therapist to charge for the cost of providing this. Yet, unfortunately, the patient usually has to pay for this and is not compensated by the insurer.

Before such information is provided, it is essential that the patient sign a release. Photocopied releases "to all medical providers" may not be valid. Familiarity with confidentiality requirements may be obtained by consulting numerous sources, including Stromberg et al. (1988) and Pope (1990).

ASSIGNMENT (SECTION E)

Box 13 "assigns" benefits so that the practitioner can be paid directly by the insurance company. Many therapists ask patients to pay their co-payment but accept assignment of the balance. For instance, if an individual has 80% coverage and has met his or her deductible, the therapist who charges $100 per session may accept $20 from the patient at the session, and $80 "on assignment" from the insurance company.

Medicare and Blue Shield allow practitioners to accept assignment only as participating providers. Participation also obligates them to accept the insurer's allowable fee as payment in full. Increasingly, private insurers are trying to contain costs by tying acceptance of assignment to acceptance of the insurer's maximum charge.

It is safest to have the *insured* authorize assignment, regardless of who is the patient. In hostile divorces, a therapist might ask the custodial parent, who is not actually the insured, to sign this box, but the insurance company has the discretion to accept or reject such authorization.

Even if therapists accept assignment of a fee determined by the insurance company, they are required to collect applicable deductibles or co-payments. For example, a participating Medicare provider might bill $110 for a psychotherapy session. If Medicare allows a $90 charge, it may pay the practitioner $45 (50%) and leave $45 as the co-payment. The practitioner should collect the remaining $45 from the patient but is forbidden from collecting the $20 difference between his or her fee and what Medicare allowed. The issue of waiving co-payments will be more fully explored in Chapter 4.

Accepting assignment assures direct payment to the practitioner. This may be especially important for those therapists treating hospital patients. These patients are frequently seen for a single consultation, or if seen in psychotherapy on a mental health unit, may not continue as outpatients. They may be confused and forget that the consultation occurred. Even when they remember the consultation, they may feel less commitment to the therapist than do most office patients. It is generally impractical to collect directly from hospital patients. Most practitioners report a larger proportion of nonpayment from hospital patients than from those seen in their offices.

Accepting assignment may also be advantageous for the patients of those practitioners who receive payment at each session. If the therapist requests only the co-payment, patients may not suffer cash flow problems and be able to continue treatment. Many patients with 50% to 80% coverage can afford the co-payments but cannot afford to wait several months before receiving reimbursement. Of course, the therapist who accepts assignment will also face a cash flow problem.

An obvious disadvantage to accepting assignment occurs in participating plans where practitioners accept less than their usual fees in exchange for assignment and other benefits of participating. Other disadvantages include not receiving immediate payment and possible collection problems if reimbursement amounts are less than anticipated or if the deductible has not been met.

DATES OF ILLNESS AND FIRST CONSULTATION (SECTION F)

The practitioner should complete the remainder of the form. Block 14 contains the date that the first symptom or accident occurred. For many psychological conditions, these dates are extremely hard to ascertain. If the condition being treated is the result of an accident, it is important to record that date. In our office, we usually leave Block 14 blank and fill in the date first consulted in Block 15.

These dates may prove very important. Most plans have clauses concerning preexisting conditions. Although some will never pay for a preexisting condition, it is more typical to deny payment on preexisting conditions for 1 to 2 years. Thus, if a patient who was receiving therapy for depression changes jobs and is covered under a different plan, the new insurance company may refuse to pay for psychotherapy for a year or more.

Block 16A is provided because emergency medical care is often reimbursed at a higher rate than regular care. This block seems to have little applicability to mental health treatment. If there is a genuine emergency, such as a suicidal crisis, and extraordinary services are performed, it would be a good idea to check this box to increase the chances that reimbursement would occur. Although the initial claims processor would probably reject the unusual charge, it might be accepted on appeal. As previously discussed, however, the time required to justify a single claim for extraordinary service may be longer than the time required to provide the actual service.

DISABILITY (SECTION G)

Blocks 17 and 18 occasionally apply to mental health practitioners. Patients with severe depression, thought disorder, agoraphobia, or other conditions may not be able to work because of their mental condition. One should be aware of the possible implications of declaring, on a signed form, that the patient is disabled and unable to work and be ready and willing to substantiate this declaration. In our office this block is usually left blank.

REFERRING PHYSICIAN (SECTION H)

Many therapists, especially those covered by Freedom of Choice statutes, become resentful when insurance companies request the name of the referring physician or other agency. It is not clear why this information is requested, but it seems within the prerogative of the insurance company to demand such data before processing a claim. Generally, it creates no problems for those entitled to reimbursement. Whether a physician, social worker, school counselor, friend, or "self" refers the patient, it should not affect reimbursement.

If the practitioner is not protected by Freedom of Choice statutes, this block becomes important. Some plans will explicitly reimburse members of a particular profession only if the patient was referred by a physician. In other cases, even if there is no official policy, counselors and other therapists may be reimbursed if the patient is referred by a physician or, occasionally, by a psychologist. We usually list only physicians, mental health practitioners, and school personnel. Otherwise we leave this block blank.

HOSPITALIZATION (SECTION I)

On claims for inpatient services, insurance companies frequently ask for admission and discharge dates, supposedly for the purpose of coordinating services and making sure that duplicate or inappropriate services are not reimbursed. Unfortunately, supplying these dates creates a major inconvenience for therapists who perform hospital consultations. When reviewing the patient's chart, the admission date is easily obtained, but the consultant rarely knows when the patient is discharged. In our office we often leave this item blank, but it has led to denied or delayed claims. Another alternative is to call the medical records department of the hospital before filing a claim, a procedure that does not endear our office to that already overworked department.

LOCATION (SECTION J)

If practitioners perform the services in their offices, Block 21 can be left blank. Otherwise, indicate the hospital, emergency room, nursing home, or the patient's home address.

Block 22 is likely to pertain only to psychiatrists and physicians. Block 22B usually does not apply to any mental health practice.

DIAGNOSIS (SECTION K)

Much has been written and discussed concerning the use of diagnoses. Most insurance companies prefer the Ninth Revision of the *International Classification of Diseases - ICD-9-CM* (World Health Organization - WHO, 1989) or the Revised Third Edition of the *Diagnostic and Statistical Manual of Mental Disorders* (*DSM-III-R*; American Psychiatric Association - APA, 1987). The *ICD-9-CM* is a clinical modification of the Ninth International Classification of Diseases, a project of the World Health Organization. The *DSM-III-R* is the fourth revision of the American Psychiatric Association's manual of mental disorders, the original having been published in 1952.

The *ICD-9-CM* and the *DSM-III-R* are similar but there are some differences. A discussion of the philosophical differences and a comparison of codes can be found in Appendix E of the *DSM-III-R*. Many nonpsychiatrists object to the use of the *DSM-III-R* or *ICD-9-CM* because they closely follow a medical model. Wiggins (1988a), a psychologist, believes the *ICD-9-CM* is "more viable" than the *DSM-III-R*. All insurance claims agents have the *ICD-9-CM* available because it classifies all medical conditions. Wiggins also believes that the *ICD-9-CM* has a "richer array of diagnoses available" and assails the revisions of the *DSM-III-R* as a "profit tool" for the American Psychiatric Association. Mental health practitioners who reject the medical model have devised various classification schemes. This activity seemed to reach its peak in the early 1970s. Whatever merit these plans have, use of anything but the *DSM-III-R* or the *ICD-9-CM* will increase the likelihood of a claims denial. Most insurance forms allow room for three diagnoses. It is unclear whether one should list every possible diagnosis or only the predominant one. Some clinicians list only Axis I diagnoses, while others also list Axis II personality disorders.

Ethical and practical issues in reporting diagnoses will be discussed in Chapter 4. It is obviously fraudulent to record an incorrect diagnosis. Nevertheless, in mental health settings, several diagnoses may be appropriate. Some patients have more than one mental illness, while many overlap more than one category.

Practitioners often fear that a severe diagnosis may have an adverse effect if the patient or others become aware of it, while an overly mild one might result in nonreimbursement. Unfortunately both of these fears may be well founded.

The *DSM-III-R* contains 14 *V codes* for conditions not attributable to a mental disorder, but which are a focus of treatment. These include academic problems, antisocial behavior, and marital, occupational, and parenting difficulties. As these are not "mental disorders," they are almost never reimbursed by medical insurance.

In our office we strive for an honest diagnosis that will be accurate, meet the patient's needs, and not mislead the insurance company. If the focus of treatment is depression or anxiety disorder, we will generally not list an underlying personality disorder. On the other hand, if a patient presents with an Axis I disorder, but treatment is complicated because of a co-existing personality disorder, we will also list that disorder. If the claim form is likely to be seen by a fellow employee, we will attempt to use the mildest accurate diagnosis. In general, because of possible lapses in confidentiality, we try to use the least stigmatizing accurate diagnosis that will insure payment. If I am treating an individual for an anxiety problem but I suspect some schizoid or paranoid personality features, or even a brief psychotic episode, I will be reluctant to list those. On the other hand, if I am treating a person with chronic schizophrenia who is also receiving antipsychotic medication from a physician, I will use the diagnosis of schizophrenia.

In Figure 1 (p. 16), Jason is an adolescent who first came to the attention of Dr. Charleston when he was admitted to the hospital, through the family physician, Dr. Fantine, because of a superficial suicidal gesture. Dr. Charleston performed a psychological consultation and diagnosed a longstanding depressive disorder. He also noted an academic problem but no learning disability. He did not believe the adolescent was acutely suicidal and thought a lengthy hospitalization would be countertherapeutic. He therefore recommended discharge and outpatient follow-up. The patient and his family agreed to this plan and continued treatment with Dr. Charleston.

Although Dr. Charleston assessed a dysthymic disorder, which met all criteria of the *DSM-III-R*, as well as academic and family problems, only the dysthymic disorder is recorded. Including academic (V62.30) and family problems (V62.20) is likely to confuse the claims processor. If there are co-existing reimbursable codes, such as mental retardation (317.00, 318.00, . . .), attention deficit hyperactivity disorder (314.01), or a personality disorder, these might be included along with the Axis I disorder.

Frequently it is better to submit separate claims for inpatient and outpatient services. In Figure 1, these were mixed to provide a more varied example. The risk of mistakes by the claims processor increases dramatically when inpatient and outpatient services are combined on the same form, resulting in delayed reimbursement and additional time on the part of the therapist's office to sort out these problems.

PROCEDURE CODES (SECTION L)

Table 1 (p. 22) lists some common procedure codes. The Fourth Edition of the physician's *Current Procedural Terminology - CPT-4* (American Medical Association, 1988) provides complete listings. A local Blue Shield office is likely to provide these, free of charge. Most private carriers accept *CPT-4* codes. Local carriers may add various codes, prefixes, or suffixes such as -WD (mental), or -75 (concurrent care, services rendered by more than one provider). Medicare has developed new codes for psychotherapy and assessment performed by nonphysicians (see Table 1).

The current example shows some possible complications. The first contact with the patient was shortly after admission, when Dr. Charleston performed a comprehensive consultation, lasting approximately 1 hour 55 minutes. At this time, the psychologist took a history, assessed the patient's current condition, met with the parents, consulted with the hospital staff, and made recommendations. Accomplishing this work in under

TABLE 1: SOME COMMON MENTAL HEALTH PROCEDURE CODES

Hospital Medical Services
90200 - Initial hospital care
90240 - Subsequent hospital care: Brief
90250 - Subsequent hospital care: Limited
90260 - Subsequent hospital care: Intermediate
90270 - Subsequent hospital care: Extended
90280 - Subsequent hospital care: Comprehensive

Initial Consultation
90600 - Limited
90605 - Intermediate
90610 - Extensive
90620 - Comprehensive
90630 - Complex

Follow-Up Consultation
90640 - Brief
90641 - Limited
90642 - Intermediate
90643 - Complex

90801 - Psychiatric diagnostic interview examination including history, mental status, or disposition
90830 - Psychological testing by physician, with written report, per hour
90831 - Telephone consultation with or about patient for psychiatric, therapeutic, or diagnostic purposes.

Individual Medical Psychotherapy
90841 - Time unspecified
90843 - Approximately 20-30 minutes
90844 - Approximately 45-50 minutes

90847 - Family medical psychotherapy
90853 - Group medical psychotherapy

Note: From *Current Procedural Terminology - CPT-4* (4th ed.) by American Medical Association, 1988, Chicago, IL: American Medical Association.

Special Medicare Codes
M0601 - Psychological testing by clinical psychologist, with written report, per hour
H5010 - Psychotherapy, individual by nonphysician, per hour
H5020 - Psychotherapy, group by nonphysician, 45-50 minutes
H5025 - Psychotherapy, group by nonphysician, 90 minutes
H5030 - Other services by nonphysician, per hour (behavior modification, hypnotherapy, consultation, client-centered advocacy, crisis intervention, information and education to clients)

2 hours was clearly not excessive, and charging for his time is appropriate. Nevertheless, the insurance company is likely to pay a far lower fee. Comprehensive Psychological/Psychiatric Consultations (90620) by psychiatrists have traditionally been approximately 1 hour, and provider profiles are based on that. Despite noting the extra time, Dr. Charleston is likely to be paid as if this were a 50- to 60-minute consultation. If it fits the criteria listed in the *CPT-4*, he could consider calling this a Complex Psychological Consultation (90630) or appealing the claim if it is rejected.

A further complication arises if a psychologist performs *psychological testing*. Frequently both nonpsychiatric physicians and psychiatrists ask psychologists to test patients. Most private insurance carriers will pay for the testing, by the hour, as long as the amount is reasonable. It is legitimate to charge for one's entire testing time, which includes administration, scoring, and write-up. Most private carriers, Medicare, and CHAMPUS will pay these charges.

Some insurance companies request details of the tests administered. Medicare specifically states that this information should *not* be provided. CHAMPUS, on the other hand, usually asks for a listing of the individual tests administered. Including this information on the initial CHAMPUS claims may avoid delay.

Some Blue Shield plans do not allow for psychological testing. If psychological testing is requested on a patient for whom the services are not covered, psychologists have several options. They may refuse to perform the testing, risking negative feelings from referral source and possibly violating hospital agreements. Psychologists may bill patients for nonreimbursed services, but are unlikely to collect in many cases.

A third option is to redefine the service. Because the codes are overlapping, similar services often can be categorized in different ways. For example, a *comprehensive consultation* (90620) involves "an in depth evaluation of a patient with a problem requiring the development and documentation of medical data . . . the establishment or verification of a plan for further investigative and/or therapeutic management and the preparation of a report" (Pennsylvania Blue Shield, 1988, p. 1-224). A psychological evaluation with a brief history, psychological testing (development and documentation of psychological data), and report is consistent with the definition of a comprehensive psychological consultation. Therefore, a psychologist can probably legitimately use that code for a consultation that includes psychological testing. The psychologist is likely, however, to be reimbursed for little more than 1 hour of time.

Psychologists, social workers, and other mental health professionals often object to the procedure codes that refer to *physician* and *medical psychotherapy*. However, this does not seem to be a problematic legal issue. Blue Shield, Medicare, CHAMPUS, and others often define "physician" to include other providers, such as psychologists and social workers. Other plans specifically refer to "providers." Much protest was heard from nonpsychiatric providers in the 1980s when psychotherapy was redefined as "medical psychotherapy." The fear that this would undermine nonphysicians' ability to receive insurance reimbursement for their services seems to have been unfounded. As long as providers do not misrepresent their credentials, the use of medical psychotherapy codes does not seem to involve fraud or deception. I know of no case in which these semantic problems have interfered with reimbursement.

Mental health hospital services are frequently provided concurrently by more than one professional. A patient may be on the service of a psychiatrist who monitors medication, while a social worker may be providing psychotherapy. It is important to coordinate billing procedures so that the claims are not rejected because of duplication of services. Most insurance companies will pay for only one psychotherapy session per day and one psychiatric/psychological consultation per hospital stay. We have found it helpful for the two practitioners to use legitimate but different series of codes. This usually requires consultation between the two practitioners or their offices to avoid duplication of services, which would result in nonpayment to the provider who is second to file the claim.

For example, a psychologist might be seeing an individual in outpatient therapy who then becomes suicidal and requires hospitalization. The patient is hospitalized on the service of a psychiatrist who monitors medication, while the psychologist continues psychotherapy sessions. The psychiatrist might bill his initial consultation as 90620 (comprehensive consultation) and use 90260 (hospital medical services-intermediate) for shorter sessions. The psychologist might use 90844 (medical psychotherapy - 45 to 50 minutes) for longer psychotherapy sessions. If both use codes in the same series (e.g., 90843 and 90844, or 90260 and 90270), even on different days, all of the claims of one of the professionals, probably the second to file, would likely be rejected.

There are many overlapping procedure codes and possible entries. Each insurance company seems to handle these differently and may not be consistent even with itself. It is important to know which codes are likely to be accepted for particular services. It is also necessary to realize that claims processors rarely have a deep understanding of all the subtleties of mental health practice; they may respond arbitrarily or inconsistently to similar claims.

Inconsistencies may be seen even within a single program. The American Psychiatric Association Office of Economic Affairs ("Survey of Medicare," 1989) surveyed 29 Medicare carriers and found that 12 would allow the 90200 series (hospital medical services) to be used for inpatient hospital psychiatric session services without limiting additional charges for other services (such as psychotherapy) provided on the same day. Eleven other carriers indicated that they would allow the 90200 series to be used only if no other psychiatric services were being provided that day. Six carriers indicated that, contrary to *CPT-4* coding instructions, the 90200 series was not appropriate for psychiatric services.

The American Psychiatric Association ("Survey of Medicare," 1989) proposed adding 10 new codes to the *CPT*, but only two, "medical psychoanalysis" and "family medical psychotherapy (with patient present)" were accepted.

In Figure 1 (p. 16), Dr. Charleston saw Jason on March 8 with both parents for 10 minutes, saw Jason alone for 30, and then met with Mr. and Mrs. Ironwood alone for 10 more minutes. He is faced with some difficulty in specifically defining his services. He might use family therapy codes such as 90812, 90815, or 90818. Some insurance companies still reject these codes, considering family therapy to be "experimental." Many practitioners consider *individual psychotherapy* to be generic, involving any legitimate psychotherapeutic activities of the therapist in treating an individual. Thus, it is at the therapist's discretion whether to see the patient alone, partially with the family, or entirely in the context of the family. As long as the therapy is geared towards an identified patient, these practitioners consider such a case to be legitimately labeled as *individual psychotherapy*.

This logic would not apply to group therapy, which is reimbursed at a lesser rate because the therapist is dealing with numerous patients at one time. Family therapy, on the other hand, is often focused upon the problems of a specific patient. The therapist is not being reimbursed by more than one patient simultaneously. Family therapists who "treat the family" and avoid "scapegoating" an "identified patient" often have great difficulty with a medical model insurance system which requires an individually identified patient and diagnosis.

In treating patients, particularly children and adolescents, it is sometimes advisable to meet separately with other family members. It can be considered an inherent part of responsible practice to meet with parents or others, perhaps out of the presence of the patient. One can code this as *collateral visit* (90887), but this designation is likely to be challenged or denied. Some practitioners therefore consider such a meeting as part of generic *individual psychotherapy*, if the purpose of the collateral visit is helping the identified patient.

Codes for such procedures as telephone consultation with or about the patient (90831), environmental intervention (i.e., consultation with employers, institutions, or others - 90882), and preparation of report (90889) are almost never reimbursed by insurance companies.

PROVIDER INFORMATION (SECTION M)

Although a signature stamp may be accepted, it is usually preferable to sign claims personally. It is important to read, often on the reverse side, exactly what is being implied by one's signature (see Figure 2, p. 26). Practitioners are vulnerable to accusations of misrepresentation and fraud, which are criminal offenses, once the claim form is signed.

In Box 31 (Figure 1), we have found it helpful also to include the therapist's license number, tax identification, and social security number. In Figure 1, the social security number or the tax identification number of the practitioner was specifically requested. Nevertheless, we receive calls almost on a weekly basis from insurers who are holding up claims processing for this information, although we have clearly provided it. A rubber stamp with all of the needed information, saves clerical time.

SUPERBILLS AND STATEMENTS

A superbill is a preprinted statement that includes most diagnoses and procedures utilized by the therapist. It provides sufficient information so that it can serve as both a receipt and an insurance claim form to be submitted by the patient. The superbill is a good option for the practitioner who prefers not to be involved in the complex clerical work of completing and filing forms. Superbills can be purchased from medical stationery firms (listed in Appendix A, pp. 87-88), individually designed, or generated by a computerized billing program. A commercially prepared superbill is illustrated in Figure 3 (p. 27), and a computer generated superbill appears in Appendix B (pp. 89-95).

This form must include all relevant information, including the practitioner's credentials, tax identification (or social security number) and license number, patient's diagnosis, date and description of services, charges, and practitioner's stamp or signature. Because mental health services and diagnoses are relatively limited, all may be printed on the form and circled.

BECAUSE THIS FORM IS USED BY VARIOUS GOVERNMENT AND PRIVATE HEALTH PROGRAMS, SEE SEPARATE INSTRUCTIONS ISSUED BY APPLICABLE PROGRAM.

REFERS TO GOVERNMENT PROGRAMS ONLY

MEDICARE AND CHAMPUS PAYMENTS: A patient's signature requests that payment be made and authorizes release of medical information necessary to pay the claim. If item 9 is completed, the patient's signature authorizes releasing of the information to the insurer or agency shown. In Medicare assigned or CHAMPUS participation cases, the physician agrees to accept the charge determination of the Medicare carrier or CHAMPUS fiscal intermediary as the full charge, and the patient is responsible only for the deductible, coinsurance, and noncovered services. Coinsurance and the deductible are based upon the charge determination of the Medicare carrier of CHAMPUS fiscal intermediary if this is less than the charge

submitted. CHAMPUS is not a health insurance program and renders payment for health benefits provided through membership and affiliation with the Uniformed Services. Information on the patient's sponsor should be provided in those items captioned ''Insured'', i.e.items 3, 6, 7, 8, 9, and 11.

BLACK LUNG AND FECA CLAIMS: The provided agrees to accept the amount paid by the Government as payment in full. See Black Lung FECA instructions regarding required procedure and diagnosis coding systems.

SIGNATURE OF PHYSICIAN OR SUPPLIER (MEDICARE, CHAMPUS, FECA AND BLACK LUNG)

I certify that the services shown on this form were medically indicated and necessary for the health of the patient and were personally rendered by me or were rendered incident to my professional service by my employee under immediate personal supervision, except as otherwise expressly permitted by Medicare or CHAMPUS regulations.

For services to be considered an 'incident' to a physician's professional service, 1) they must be rendered under the physician's immediate personal supervision by his/her employee, 2) they must be an integral,

although incidental part of a covered physician's service, 3) they must be of kinds commonly furnished in physician's offices, and 4) the services of nonphysicians must be included on the physician's bills.

For CHAMPUS claims, I further certify that neither I nor any employee who rendered the services are employees or members of the Uniformed Services (refer to 5 USC 5536). For Black-Lung claims, I further certify that the services performed were for a Black Lung related disorder.

No Part B Medicare benefits may be paid unless this form is received as required by existing law and regulations (20 CFR 422 510).

NOTICE: Any one who misrepresents or falsifies essential information to receive payment from Federal funds requested by this form may upon conviction be subject to fine and imprisonment under applicable Federal laws.

NOTICE TO PATIENT ABOUT THE COLLECTION AND USE OF MEDICARE, CHAMPUS, FECA, AND BLACK LUNG INFORMATION

We are authorized by HCFA, CHAMPUS and OWCP to ask you for information needed in the administration of the Medicare, CHAMPUS, FECA, and BLACK LUNG programs. Authority to collect information is in section 205 (a), 1872 and 1875 of the Social Security Act as amended and 44 USC 3101, 41 CFR 101 et seq and 10 USC 1079 and 1086; 5 USC 8101 et seq; and 30 USC 901 et seq.

The information we obtain to complete claims under these programs is used to identify you and to determine your eligibility. It is also used to decide if the services and supplies you received are covered by these programs and to insure that proper payment is made.

The information may also be given to other providers of services, carriers, intermediaries, medical review boards and other organizations or

Federal agencies as necessary to administer these programs. For example, it may be necessary to disclose information about the benefits you have used to a hospital or doctor.

With the one exception discussed below, there are no penalties under these programs for refusing to supply information. However, failure to furnish information regarding the medical services rendered or the amount charged would prevent payment of claims under these programs. Failure to furnish any other information, such as name or claim number, would delay payment of the claim.

It is mandatory that you tell us if you are being treated for a work related injury so we can determine whether workers' compensation will pay for treatment. Section 1877 (a) (3) of the Social Security Act provides criminal penalties for withholding this information.

MEDICAID PAYMENTS (PROVIDER CERTIFICATION)

I hereby agree to keep such records as are necessary to disclose fully the extent of services provided to individuals under the State's Title XIX plan and to furnish information regarding any payments claimed for providing such services as the State Agency or Dept. of Health and Human Services may request. I further agree to accept, as payment in full the amount paid by the Medicaid program for those claims submitted for payment under that program, with the exception of authorized deductibles and coinsurance.

SIGNATURE OF PHYSICIAN (OR SUPPLIER): I certify that the services listed above were medically indicated and necessary to the health of this patient and were personally rendered by me or my employee under my personal direction.

NOTICE: This is to certify that the foregoing information is true, accurate and complete.

I understand that payment and satisfaction of this claim will be from Federal and/or State funds, and that any false claims, statements, or documents or concealment of a material fact, may be prosecuted under applicable Federal or State laws.

PLACE OF SERVICE CODES:
1 - (IH) - Inpatient Hospital
2 - (OH) - Outpatient Hospital
3 - (O) - Doctor's Office
4 - (H) - Patient's Home
5 - - Day Care Facility (PSY)
6 - - Night Care Facility (PSY)
7 - (NH) - Nursing Home
8 - (SNF) - Skilled Nursing Facility
9 - - Ambulance
0 - (OL) - Other Locations
A - (IL) - Independent Laboratory
B - (ASC) - Ambulatory Surgical Center
C - (RTC) - Residential Treatment Center
D - (STF) - Specialized Treatment Facility
E - (COR) - Comprehensive Outpatient Rehabilitation Facility
F - (KDC) - Independent Kidney Disease Treatment Center

TYPE OF SERVICE CODES:
1 - Medical Care
2 - Surgery
3 - Consultation
4 - Diagnostic X-Ray
5 - Diagnostic Laboratory
6 - Radiation Therapy
7 - Anesthesia
8 - Assistance at Surgery
9 - Other Medical Service
0 - Blood or Packed Red Cells
A - Used DME
F - Ambulatory Surgical Center
H - Hospice
L - Renal Supplies in the Home
M - Alternate Payment for Maintenance Dialysis
N - Kidney Donor
V - Pneumococcal Vaccine
Y - Second Opinion on Elective Surgery
Z - Third Opinion on Elective Surgery

Note. Reprinted with permission of Colwell Systems, Inc., P.O. Box 4024, Champaign, Illinois 61824-4024.

Figure 2. Health Insurance Claim Form - Reverse Side.

YOUR NAME, Degree
Corporation Name
Specialty Designation
Street Address, Suite #
City, State and Zip
Area Code and Phone Number
License (number, state, type)
Tax ID or Social Security #
Other Information (Board Certification, National Register, etc.)

SERVICES BILLED TO

PATIENT INFORMATION		
POLICY HOLDER		
SOCIAL SECURITY NUMBER		
STREET		
CITY	STATE	ZIP
PATIENT John Doe		☒ MALE ☐ FEMALE
PATIENT'S BIRTHDATE		
MONTH	DAY	YEAR
INSURANCE CARRIER		
POLICY NO.	GROUP NO.	
RELATIONSHIP TO POLICY HOLDER		

*NOTICE TO INSURED
1. Complete patient information section.
2. Sign and date.
3. Retain one copy for your records.
4. Send one copy to your insurance company.

AUTHORIZATION TO RELEASE INFORMATION
I hereby authorize the release of any information acquired in the course of my examination and treatment.

Signature_____
(Patient or parent if minor.)

Date_____

AUTHORIZATION TO ASSIGN BENEFITS
I certify that the services listed have been received and I authorize payment to be made directly to said clinician.

Signature_____
(Patient or parent if minor.)

Date_____

DIAGNOSIS CODES	
DISRUPTIVE BEHAVIOR DISORDERS	
314.01	Attention-deficit dis
312.20	Conduct dis; group type
312.00	solitary agg type
312.90	undiff type
EATING DISORDERS	
307.10	Anorexia nervosa
307.51	Bulimia nervosa
ELIMINATION DISORDERS	
307.70	Functional encopresis
307.60	Functional enuresis
ORGANIC MENTAL DISORDERS	
Dementia, Alzh type	
290.30	Senile onset w/ delirium
290.20	w/ delusions
290.21	w/ depression
290.00	uncomplicated
290.1	Presenile onset
290.4	Multi-infarct dementia
SUBSTANCE USE DISORDERS	
303.90	Alcohol, dep
305.00	abuse
304.40	Amphetamine, dep
305.70	abuse
304.30	Cannabis, dep
305.20	abuse
304.20	Cocaine, dep
305.60	abuse
304.50	Hallucinogen, dep
305.30	abuse
304.60	Inhalant, dep
305.90	abuse
305.10	Nicotine, dep
304.00	Opioid, dep
305.50	abuse
304.50	Phencyclidine, dep
305.90	abuse
304.10	Sed, hypn, or anxio, dep
305.40	abuse
304.90	Polysubstance dep
SCHIZOPHRENIA	
295.2	Catatonic
295.1	Disorganized
295.3	Paranoid
295.9	Undifferentiated
295.6	Residual
OTHER PSYCHOTIC DISORDERS	
298.80	Brief reactive psychosis
295.40	Schizophreniform dis
295.70	Schizoaffective dis
297.30	Induced psychotic dis
MOOD DISORDERS	
296.6	Bipolar, mixed
296.4	manic
296.5	depressed
301.13	Cyclothymia
296.2	Major depression, sgl epis
296.3	recurrent
300.40	Dysthymia
ANXIETY DISORDERS	
300.21	Panic dis, w/agoraphobia
300.01	w/o agoraphobia
300.22	Agoraphobia, w/o panic dis
300.23	Social phobia

300.29	Simple phobia
300.30	Obs/comp dis
309.89	Post-traumatic stress dis
300.02	Generalized anxiety dis
SOMATOFORM DISORDERS	
300.11	Conversion dis
300.70	Hypochondriasis
300.81	Somatization dis
307.80	Somatoform pain dis
300.70	Undiff somatoform dis
DISSOCIATIVE DISORDERS	
300.14	Multiple personality dis
300.13	Psychogenic fugue
300.12	Psychogenic amnesia
300.60	Depersonalization dis
SEXUAL DISORDERS	
302.40	Exhibitionism
302.81	Fetishism
302.20	Pedophilia
302.83	Sexual masochism
302.84	Sexual sadism
302.82	Voyeurism
302.75	Premature ejaculation
306.51	Vaginismus
SLEEP DISORDERS	
307.42	Insomnia dis, non-organic
780.50	organic
307.42	Primary insomnia
307.47	Dream anxiety dis
307.46	Sleep terror dis
307.46	Sleepwalking dis
FACTITIOUS DISORDERS	
301.51	w/ phys symptoms
300.16	w/ psych symptoms
IMPULSE CONTROL DISORDERS	
312.34	Intermittent expl dis
312.32	Kleptomania
312.31	Pathological gambling
312.33	Pyromania
312.39	Trichotillomania
ADJUSTMENT DISORDER	
309.24	w/ anxious mood
309.00	w/ depressed mood
309.30	w/ disturb of conduct
309.40	w/ mixed disturb of emot/cond
309.28	w/ mixed emot feat
309.82	w/ physical complaints
309.83	w/ withdrawal
309.23	w/ work/acad inhibition
PSY FACTORS AFFECTING PHYS COND	
316.00	Psy factors affecting a phys cond
PERSONALITY DISORDERS	
301.00	Paranoid
301.20	Schizoid
301.22	Schizotypal
301.70	Antisocial
301.83	Borderline
301.50	Histrionic
301.81	Narcissistic
301.82	Avoidant
301.60	Dependent

301.40	Obsessive compulsive
301.84	Passive aggressive
OTHER DIAGNOSIS	

PROCEDURE CODES	
HOSPITAL CARE	
90200	Brief hist and exam
90215	Intermediate hist and exam
90220	Comprehensive hist & exam
90240	Each day; brief srvcs
90250	limited srvcs
90260	intermediate srvcs
90270	extended srvcs
90280	comprehensive srvcs
90292	Hospital discharge
THERAPEUTIC INJECTIONS	
90782	Injection of medication
	Specify:
90784	Intravenous
INTERVIEW PROCEDURES	
90801	Diagnostic interview exam
90825	Evaluation tech'l or rpts
90830	Psychological testing
90833	Telephone consultation
90835	Narcosynthesis
THERAPEUTIC PROCEDURES	
90841	Indiv psychotherapy; unspec
90843	20-30 min
90844	45-50 min
90847	Family psychotherapy
90849	Mult fam grp psychotherapy
90853	Group psychotherapy
90870	ECT; single seizure
90871	mult seizures per day
90880	Hypnotherapy
90882	Environmental intervention
90887	Interpret of exam results
90889	Preparation of report
90899	Unlisted procedure
BIOFEEDBACK	
90900	Biofeedback training
90904	reg of blood pressure
90906	reg of skin temp
90908	by EEG application
MEDICAL PROCEDURE CODES	
Office Visits	
90020	Init. Comprehensive eval
90060	Intermediate visit
90070	Extended visit
Hospital Consultations	
90620	Initial, comprehensive
90630	Initial, complex
90643	Follow-up
UNCODED PROCEDURES	
	Missed appointment
	Court appearance
	Divorce mediation
	Supervision
	Other (specify)
LOCATION	
	Office
	Hospital
	Other

SAMPLE
DO NOT USE

DATES	
Jan. 3, 10, 17, 24, 31 1990	
Service ____ Diagnosis ____	
Total Sessions 5	Charge Per Session 90.00

TOTAL CHARGES
450.00

ADJUSTMENTS

PAYMENTS
200.00

PRIOR BALANCE

LATE CHARGES

☐ BALANCE
DELINQUENT IF CHECKED

BALANCE DUE ▶ 250.00

x *Your name, degree*
PROVIDER'S SIGNATURE

© SUPER ᴪ BILL BY THE OVERHEADSHRINKERS REV. (7/89) (818) 799-6882

Note. Reprinted with permission of The Overheadshrinkers, P.O. Box 3677, South Pasadena, California 91031.

Figure 3. Sample Superbill.

The practitioner may also use a standard invoice or statement form (see Figures 4 and 5, pp. 30-31). Patients can attach these statements to the insurance forms they submit to their insurance companies. With word processing, the therapist's office can prepare the format so that only the specific details for an individual patient need to be entered.

In our office, we do not limit the number of statements we provide or forms we will complete. Unlike a family medical practice, which may provide services to 10 or more patients per hour, our actual clerical cost for complying with these requests is relatively low. Although it requires time and is sometimes frustrating, we collect approximately 99% of our office fees. We believe this reflects patients' satisfaction with both the therapeutic and the administrative and clerical services of our office. We consider clerical costs, lost interest (due to delays of 2 to 12 weeks and occasionally much longer, in receiving reimbursement from insurance companies), completing forms, and billing patients to be minor overhead expenses. Very few of our uncollectible accounts could be prevented by different billing or insurance procedures. Many of the lost fees come from patients who come one time, "forget" their checkbooks, and never return.

FILING CLAIMS

In dealing with insurance, what seems obvious often is not. For instance, the address to which claims are to be sent is frequently absent from the form. Claims may be mailed to the employer or directly to the insurance company. Responses and/or checks frequently come from regions of the country that are different from the address to which the original claim was submitted. Thus, it is always essential to determine exactly where to send the claim and, if questions arise, where to direct inquiries.

The frequency of filing insurance forms varies with the inclination of the patient and therapist, as well as particular requirements of the plan. When my office assumes the responsibility, we file no more frequently than monthly. Therapists with computerized billing systems may file weekly or even daily. Some patients prefer to accumulate several months' worth of sessions before filing. Most insurance companies require claims to be filed within a specific period. Claims may be invalid if filed more than 1 year after the date of service. Other companies require claims to be filed within 90 days of the service, or perhaps 90 days after the end of the year. Some insurance companies request that no claim be made until a specific number of sessions has occurred or termination of treatment, whichever comes first.

One problem is the tendency of some insurance companies to delay responding to claims for months, despite state laws which mandate action within specified timeframes (usually 30 days). Some practitioners report that claims are paid faster when they stamp all insurance claim forms and envelopes with the following imprint:

> Unless this claim is paid or denied within
> 30 days, we will file a formal complaint
> with the Insurance Commissioner.

If therapists warn insurance companies of such a standard procedure (i.e., filing formal complaints after 30 days), they will be obligated to generally follow through. Such complaints could be filed with a simple form letter.

REJECTED CLAIMS

Often insurance companies reject claims for legitimate reasons. The insurance policy may not have been in effect when the service was delivered. The patient's coverage may not have included mental health benefits; or it may have excluded preexisting conditions. The patient may not have met the deductible or may have exceeded a maximum benefit. The form may have been incomplete, or an incorrect form may have been submitted.

Other legitimate, though controversial, reasons for rejection include circumstances wherein the employer is self-insured or the policy is written out of the state and covered by different rules. These situations will be discussed later.

The most common illegitimate reason for denying a claim is a clerical error. Commonly, the claims processor has misread or misentered the place of service (perhaps reimbursement for inpatient services was only 50%, the amount appropriate for outpatient services), the amount of time on psychological testing, or a procedure code. Sometimes a claims processor makes a judgmental error (e.g., not realizing that non-physicians are eligible for reimbursement in that particular state, or that the MMPI is a psychological test). We have found that claims on which the length of session is not precisely specified are often rejected. On each claim, we list not only the procedure code, but a description of the type and length of service (e.g., 90844 - psychotherapy - full).

These errors are usually easy to correct. The practitioner may devise an appeal form or merely send a letter. One should include the subscriber's identification and group numbers, the claim number, and the reason for appeal. It is helpful to include a copy of the rejected claim, and the actual written response form from the insurance company.

We have had a particular problem with Medicare, which reimburses psychological testing on a *per-hour* basis. We have tried to highlight the amount of testing time by underlining, highlighting in pink or blue, and circling in asterisks. Yet our Medicare carrier usually initially reimburses for only 1 hour of testing. We have a standard letter prepared on the word processor, in which we insert the patient's name, control numbers, and date of testing (Figure 6, p. 32).

Several weeks after sending this letter, we usually receive the proper reimbursement. Despite the inconvenience and delay in reimbursement, we continue to file these forms and follow-up letters because the alternative of trying to change a bureaucracy is a daunting prospect.

Occasionally, appeals on legitimate claims are also rejected or ignored. It is then helpful to write a follow-up letter, perhaps with documentation, such as a copy of the state's Freedom of Choice Law or the patient's benefits manual. This can be done by the practitioner or the patient. If the insurance company is clearly in violation of its policy or the law, this can be appealed to the state insurance commissioner. At that time, it would also be helpful to contact the therapist's state professional organization

RICHARD F. SMALL, PH.D.
CLINICAL PSYCHOLOGIST
122 WEST LANCASTER AVENUE
SHILLINGTON, PA 19607

(215) 777-6868
PENNSYLVANIA LICENSE # PS-002912-L

KERRY KLINGER, A.T., M.S.   ANTOINETTE WISWESSER, R.N.C.

Mr. and Mrs. Sanford Shirley
1620 Joseph Avenue
Wheatland, KS 67000

FOR PROFESSIONAL SERVICES: Evelyn Shirley
                             Dx: 309.28 (DSM III-R)
July 11 - Psychotherapy $100.00
July 15 - Psychological testing - CBCL   60.00
July 18 - Psychological testing - 1½ hr. 150.00
July 25 - Psychotherapy (consultation
          with parents)   100.00

          Balance due $410.00

July 26, 1991

ALL CLINICAL SERVICES ARE PERFORMED DIRECTLY BY,
OR UNDER THE SUPERVISION OF RICHARD F. SMALL, PH.D.

Figure 4. Sample Invoice.

RICHARD F. SMALL, PH.D.
CLINICAL PSYCHOLOGIST
122 WEST LANCASTER AVENUE
SHILLINGTON, PA 19607
(215) 777-6868

Lee A. Bergen
1991 Statement
Dx: 300.40 (DSM III-R)

May 2 - Psychotherapy	$100.00
May 9 - Psychotherapy	100.00
May 13 - Psychological testing - MMPI	50.00
May 16 - Psychotherapy	100.00
May 23 - Psychotherapy	100.00
May 30 - Psychotherapy	100.00
June 6 - Psychotherapy	100.00
June 13 - Psychotherapy	100.00
June 20 - Psychotherapy	100.00

All sessions were full sessions of fifty
minutes.

Tax ID # 23-2083419
PA License # PS 002912L

June 22, 1991

> All clinical services are performed
> directly by, or under the supervision
> of Richard F. Small, Ph.D.

Figure 5. Sample Statement.

RICHARD F. SMALL, PH.D.
CLINICAL PSYCHOLOGIST
122 WEST LANCASTER AVENUE
SHILLINGTON, PA 19607
(215) 777-6868

January 4, 1991

Medicare
P.O. Box 65
Camp Hill, PA 17011

To Whom It May Concern:

I am writing regarding Deborah Rachelwitz, claim number, 194237026, control number 70923654321. The claim was filed for psychological testing, 2 hours. The reimbursement you approved was what has customarily been paid for psychological testing, per hour. I believe that the reimbursement was erroneous. Your immediate attention to this matter will be appreciated.

Sincerely,

Richard F. Small, Ph.D.

RFS:mss

Figure 6. Sample Letter to Medicare.

(psychiatric society, psychological association, etc.) for information and possible support in an appeal.

Sometimes rejections that fall into a gray area, or even those that are legitimate, can be appealed. I have heard of many therapists, not covered by Freedom of Choice laws, or where policies clearly do not include a particular service, whose claims were first rejected, but upon appeal, quietly paid. Insurance companies may elect to make reimbursement, but do not want to publicly set a precedent.

Other pressures can sometimes be applied, which may change insurance companies' policies. Most mental health coverage is limited because many people do not expect to need it, and if they do, are embarrassed to assert themselves. Yet as the stigma of receiving mental health services decreases, we hope more patients will be willing to request such coverage.

Patients may also be willing to inform their employers of the inadequate mental health coverage. It is ethically imperative to warn patients of the possible consequences of their actions and to be sure that they are not being used for the therapist's purposes. Nevertheless, it may be appropriate, and even therapeutic, for a patient to proceed in that direction. If so, dissatisfied employees make employers aware of the inadequacies of coverage. Insurance companies are very responsive to employers' demands. Inadequate mental health coverage comes from the insurance companies' desire to please the employers with lower premiums. Insurance companies are usually happy to provide any extra coverage for which the employer is willing to pay.

COMPUTERS AND PRACTICE MANAGEMENT SOFTWARE

Many mental health professionals report that available software greatly simplifies submission of patient statements and insurance claims. When installed on an IBM PC-compatible computer, such software will allow you to:

1. Print superbills, patient statements, and insurance claims on demand (i.e., at the end of an appointment, weekly, monthly, or annually). Numerous options for formatting claims and statements are available. At least one software program (Mental Health Office Manager - MHOM) optionally allows electronic submission of claims to the carrier utilizing a modem; it has been suggested that electronic submissions of Blue Shield and Medicare claims speed payment and decrease the probability of processing errors.

2. Automate the process of recording and retrieving client information (including all relevant insurance data for both primary and secondary insurance carriers), diagnostic codes (*ICD-9-CM, DSM-III-R,* or custom codes), services (using *CPT-4* or custom codes), charges, payments (including source of payment), and adjustments. If you desire, these programs will compute finance charges and will print special notices on overdue accounts. They also track "insurance satisfaction" (exactly which sessions/claims have been paid), patient insurance deductibles, and the percentage or fixed amounts that the client owes for each session

(allowing you to bill clients for only the amount that you anticipate will not be paid by their insurance).

3. Print on demand a multitude of financial reports including unpaid accounts (accounts-aging information), reports on all services and changes for each provider, and complete tracking reports on unpaid insurance claims (by insurance carrier with notes on who to contact to facilitate payment). Some software also permits customized reports utilizing any of the information in your database.

Appendix A (pp. 87-88) provides a listing of some of the better known suppliers of software for managing a mental health practice. All of these suppliers should be able to provide you with descriptive information, low cost disks that demonstrate their programs, and reference lists of current users. Appendix B (pp. 89-95) contains samples of computer-generated forms and reports.

The major advantage of computers is speed and efficiency. Yet there are trade-offs in converting to computers. If you or your staff are not experienced in using computers, it may take some time to become familiar with the overall operation of both hardware and software. Even for experienced users, it frequently takes several weeks to gain proficiency with new software. During the transition, one might want concurrently to use the old bookkeeping system. Only after the transition is completed (often 3 to 6 months) will the benefits of computerization be obvious.

Another difficulty may be the inability to customize the computer program to exactly match your needs. Few practices can afford to hire programmers to design and customize a program to their precise specifications, so most usually select commercially prepared mental health office management software. Although the best of these programs provide many options, practitioners may have idiosyncratic needs that cannot be met by such generic software. Furthermore, as computers make decisions by logical rules (e.g., sending a past-due statement to all accounts every 30 days), it is sometimes difficult to program the computer to make individual exceptions (e.g., "This patient sometimes gets a little behind, but I know he's reliable and I don't want to offend him with a past-due statement"). Thus, a practitioner must decide whether the size of the practice and the loss of subtle decision-making options are worth the potentially increased convenience of computerization.

CHAPTER 4
LEGAL AND ETHICAL ISSUES

A great deal has been written about certain practices such as waiving co-payments, "signing off" for unlicensed therapists, and various other billing practices. The ethics of some situations are clear, but others remain murky.

It is necessary for the reader to continue to keep in mind the nature of the insurance contract. The insurance company agrees to pay for certain services, under specific circumstances, as defined in the contract. No matter how clinically appropriate, socially worthwhile, and/or ultimately cost-effective the clinician's intervention may be, the insurance company has no obligation to pay if the particular service in question is not covered in the insurance contract.

Practitioners frequently accuse insurance companies of "practicing without a license" in determining what is clinically or medically appropriate. Insurance companies reply that they are not determining what a therapist should do, but only deciding what services the insurance will cover. As a practical matter, insurance payments often do affect the therapeutic services provided. Unfortunately, insurance companies also seem to have sound legal footing when they decide what services they will cover. It is also important to realize that an insurance company's refusal to pay for services does not abrogate the therapist's ethical and legal responsibility to provide appropriate treatment.

The terms of the contract are determined by the parties (often the insurance company and employer), but are also subject to state and federal law. States can require that insurance contracts guarantee psychologists, social workers, and others eligibility for reimbursement, or that certain mental health services be covered by insurance contracts. Government plans such as Medicare, Medical Assistance, and CHAMPUS are designed by law rather than by contract negotiations.

Writers in a variety of mental health specialties have set numerous guidelines and suggestions, but all agree with Christensen (1989), who suggests "play it straight in insurance billing."

WAIVING CO-PAYMENTS, REDUCING FEES, AND OFFERING PROFESSIONAL COURTESIES

Most mental health plans require patient co-payments between 20% and 50%. Some practitioners inappropriately adjust their fees depending on a patient's insurance. In a hypothetical situation, Nelson Niceguy is a social worker in a state without a social work Freedom of Choice law. About half of his patients have no insurance coverage for his services, while the other half are covered by plans which reimburse social workers. For uninsured patients, Mr. Niceguy charges $80 per hour. For those with 80% coverage, he charges $100 per hour, so that he will receive the same $80 and the patient will not be "inconvenienced" by having to pay $20 out of pocket. For those patients with 50% coverage, he charges $160, and again does not charge a co-payment if the insurance company pays $80. If an insurance company will not pay the full $80 (e.g., if they will only pay 50% of an allowable $120 which is $60), he will charge the patient the difference between what the insurance company has paid and his $80 fee.

This practice is considered unacceptable and may be legally fraudulent (Canter & Freudenberger, 1990; Christensen, 1989; "Insurance Information," 1988; Kovacs, 1987a; "Legal Issues," 1989; Rofsky, 1989; Stromberg et al., 1988). It is unacceptable because Mr. Niceguy misrepresented the fee to the insurance carrier, which has only agreed to pay 50% or 80% of the therapist's *actual* fee. Some therapists feel that such billing practices help their poor, downtrodden patients deal with giant, impersonal, uncaring corporations, but in fact, they may be illegally committing fraud.

A practitioner must make a good-faith effort to collect co-payments. If reasonable efforts are made but fail, the practitioner has acted ethically by stating the full fee on the insurance form.

There is unanimous agreement that routine *forgiveness* of co-payments is unacceptable. Whether it is actually illegal depends on state laws, specific insurance contracts, and federal regulations. CHAMPUS specifically declares, in a section on "Fraud and Abuse," that "inflating charges to offset waiver of deductibles and cost shares" ("Office of Civilian," p. 52) is an example of abuse. Health Care Financing Administration (HCFA) regulations state that, for Medicare providers, it is not acceptable to discount services by not attempting to collect co-payment deductibles. Providers are not required to attempt to collect when the amounts are so small that the cost of collecting and billing exceeds the charge or when the provider determines the patient to be "indigent" (Pennsylvania Blue Shield, 1990).

Psychotherapy Finances ("You Could Be Jailed," 1989) reports that Houston hospitals were advertising a willingness to accept insurance company payments and to waive the usual patient co-payment. Prudential had complained to hospital administrators but never threatened the kind of legal actions which have occasionally been taken against therapists. It will be interesting to see if the illegality of routine co-payment waiver is eventually tested in court.

It may be acceptable to waive a co-payment occasionally, either as a professional courtesy or to help a needy patient. Insurance companies have privately informed therapists that this practice is permissible. Pennsylvania Blue Shield (1990), acting as

Medicare administrator, warns that if "you *routinely* [author's italics] waive a Medicare patient's deductible and co-insurance, we may reduce your actual charge" (p. 6); this language seems to imply the acceptability of an occasional waiver.

Sliding scales and reduced fees present a different problem. Sliding scales, based on a patient's income or ability to pay, have been the backbone of the public mental health system and have often been carried into private practice. On the other hand, sliding scales are unusual in medicine, which is the foundation of the health insurance system. Insurance carriers have difficulty recognizing and dealing appropriately with this fee philosophy.

As long as practitioners do not misrepresent their fees, sliding scales are permissible. Dr. Shrink is entitled to establish the following fee schedule: If income is $50,000 or more the fee is $100; for incomes of $25,000 to $50,000 the fee is $75; for patients earning less than $25,000, she charges $50. If Dr. Shrink sees a patient who has no insurance and makes $20,000, she would charge $50. If she sees a patient who earns $20,000 and has 80% insurance coverage under his insurance plan, Dr. Shrink must still charge $50, $40 coming from the insurance company and $10 from the patient. She cannot charge the insured patient her full fee of $100 just because that individual has insurance.

A further problem with a sliding scale is that it affects the practitioner's profile. Many insurance companies base their reimbursement on UCR, which includes the practitioner's *usual* fee. If Dr. Shrink is seeing many low-income people at $50 per session, a fair number of middle-income individuals at $75 and few high-income patients at $100 per hour, insurance companies are likely to record her *usual* fee as $50 or $75. If she sees a high-income patient with 80% insurance, the insurance company will probably accept only 80% of $75, or perhaps 80% of $50, considering this to be her *usual* fee. Although seemingly benevolent and humanistic, a routine sliding scale may actually reduce the therapist's reimbursement on all patients.

It is clearly appropriate and ethical to occasionally reduce fees for patients. Such exceptions may be due to a patient's change in circumstances (e.g., divorce, change of job) during the course of therapy, or as the result of a decision at the outset to see a particular patient for a lower fee. One must still report the actual fee, not the potential full fee, on insurance claims. As long as the practice is occasional, it should not seriously affect the practitioner's profile. To make it clear that this is a special fee, the practitioner might report the service on the insurance form as follows:

Psychotherapy - 1 hour	$100
Adjustment	($40)
Net fee	$60

ASSISTANTS AND SUPERVISEES

Perhaps the most scandalous and widespread practice among mental health professionals is "signing off" unlicensed therapists. Some practitioners will charge a flat amount, others a per-patient "kickback" fee, and some "sign off" as a favor for a friend with no remuneration. In any case, practitioners who sign insurance forms for services that they did not perform or truly supervise are engaging in an unethical and fraudulent practice.

In fact, both the therapist and supervisee could find themselves liable. *Psychotherapy Finances* ("Legal Briefing," 1987) reports that a licensed clinical social worker in Kentucky received a referral from a psychiatrist who continued to sign the bills that went to the insurance company. Blue Cross and Blue Shield of Kentucky pressed felony charges of theft by deception against only the social worker, who agreed to plead guilty to a misdemeanor. She was sentenced to a weekend in jail, 720 hours of community services, and 5 years of probation, and had to pay $37,000 back to Blue Cross and Blue Shield. The psychiatrist was not charged by the State's Attorney, but the Board of Medical Licensing charged him with dishonorable, unethical, or unprofessional conduct.

Although it is clearly poor practice, unethical, and probably illegal to sign forms for other therapists, the proper procedure for legitimate assistants and supervisees is less obvious. "Common wisdom" dictates that if the service is being performed by a psychological assistant, intern, or other unlicensed person, it is necessary to indicate clearly who actually provided the service (Ethics Committee of the American Psychological Association, 1988; Harran, VandeCreek, & Knapp, 1990; Maryland Psychological Association, 1990; Nagle, 1989; Tennessee Psychological Association, 1988). Most writers making this assertion accept this principle as a given. Kovacs (1987a) attacks the unethical practice of signing insurance claim forms for nonlicensed providers with whom the licensed practitioner "had no former relationship whatsoever other than that of charging for their service of filling out fraudulent claims forms" (p. 23).

Kovacs objects to insurance companies' refusal to reimburse psychological services provided by a supervisee but advises that a psychologist who "cares about steering a prudent course" will clearly identify the actual provider of the service for which the licensed professional is signing. It seems that he does not consider providing services by a supervised employee to be unethical, but advises against doing anything that could be considered misrepresentation.

Although it is illegal to intentionally mislead an insurance company into believing the services were directly performed by the supervisor, what constitutes supervision is less obvious. Health insurance is based on a traditional medical model in which the physician is responsible for all services provided by himself or herself and his or her auxiliary staff. If a patient receives an injection, or has wax cleaned out of his or her ear, these may be administered by the nurse, out of the doctor's direct presence. Nevertheless these services are properly billed under the doctor's name with no mention of the specific individual who provided the service. The doctor clearly accepts professional responsibility and, if something goes wrong, would be held liable. A similar perspective might be applied to *bona fide* supervised psychotherapeutic services.

In fact, Medicare (Nationwide Mutual Insurance Company, 1987) specifically provides for "incident to" services, provided by the nonlicensed therapist working under a licensed provider's supervision. In 1987, when this bulletin was written, only physicians were licensed providers. Since Medicare now includes psychologists and social workers as eligible providers, one can reasonably consider what applies to physicians to extend to all qualified providers. In fact, HCFA is currently developing similar "incident to" regulations for nonphysician providers.

Medicare states that, in order for "incident to" services to be reimbursed, the physician must be "actively involved in and professionally responsible for" the patient's care. This requires that:

1) "The physician must first render a covered personal professional service for which the services of the non-physician can be considered incidental, although an integral part." [The psychotherapeutic service must be one that is eligible for Medicare reimbursement and would exclude services such as those for personal growth.]

2) "The non-physician's service must be appropriate rather than a procedure which would be reserved for the physician." [The therapist should not be prescribing medicine. A non-psychologist assistant should not be providing psychological testing.]

3) "Qualified therapists may perform psychotherapy as long as there is evidence of collaborative development of a plan of treatment by the physician and therapist." [The licensed provider must be an involved supervisor.]

4) "The physician must be present in the office suite and immediately available to provide assistance and direction throughout the time the non-physician is providing the services." [The supervisor must be continually available for emergency intervention, but need not be in the therapy room.]

5) "Physician's personal, professional service must be frequent enough to assess the course of treatment and the patient's progress." [Once again, this emphasizes that the licensed provider must be involved in *bona fide* supervision.] (All quotes from Nationwide Insurance Company, 1987, pp. 1-2. Author's interpretations are in brackets.)

"Professionally responsible" also seems to indicate that the licensed provider is "administratively responsible" for the service. The supervisor must have the ability to countermand or redirect the therapist if the supervisor deems it necessary. Supervision is not merely consultation. "Professionally responsible" might include having the therapist as employee, or being in a supervisory position in an agency.

As of August, 1990, HCFA specifically indicated that "services and supplies furnished 'incident to' a CP's [clinical psychologist's] services are covered" (U.S. Department of Health & Human Services, 1990). The regulations state that the same "incident to" requirements apply to clinical psychologists and physicians. These regulations specifically require that the supervisee be an employee.

An important feature of the Medicare bulletin is the statement that "the name of the non-physician who rendered the services should *not* [Medicare's italics] be indicated on the claim. Only the name of the physician billing for the services is required" (Nationwide Insurance Company, 1987, p. 2). Thus, despite the accumulation of common wisdom that it is always inappropriate to omit the name of the therapist, Medicare has clearly stated that it is inappropriate to name the supervisee who performed the service, and is appropriate only to name the responsible provider.

Pennsylvania Blue Shield (1989b) specifically discusses mental health services "reported by one professional provider but actually performed by another" (p. 5), including psychiatric aides and psychiatric social workers. They indicate that the services are covered if they are under the provider's "direct personal supervision," which means that the provider must be in the "immediate vicinity" and be available to assist personally or assume primary care if necessary. Telephone access is specifically excluded.

Pennsylvania Blue Shield is less clear about how services should be reported, noting only that "providers should not report services they have not performed or personally supervised" (p. 5).

Kovacs (personal communication, August 14, 1990) concedes that using Medicare's position on "incident to" guidelines and not stating the exact name and title of the therapist may be legal, but he still questions the ethics of doing so.

It is also helpful to consider what is stated on the back of a standard HCFA - 1500A form (see p. 26). For Medicare and CHAMPUS, one's signature implies that "I certify that the services shown on this form were medically indicated and necessary for the health of the patient and were personally rendered by me or were rendered incident to my professional service by my employee under my immediate personal supervision, except as otherwise expressly permitted by Medicare or CHAMPUS regulations." Similarly Pennsylvania Blue Shield forms state that one's signature implies "I certify that the services reported on this form were medically necessary for the patient and were performed by me personally or in my presence, or were performed under my supervision by my employee. If the services were performed under my supervision by someone *other than my employee* [author's italics] I have described the circumstances in Item 24D."

Therefore, it seems as if it may be ethical and in keeping with acceptable insurance procedure to identify the supervisor, rather than the supervised therapist, if the former is truly "actively involved and professionally responsible" for the services. Definitions of supervision for insurance purposes may be different from requirements regarding supervision for state licensing, such as 1 hour of supervision for 4 therapy hours. Supervision for insurance clearly requires administrative responsibility as opposed to a collegial consultation relationship. It probably requires that the supervisor be physically available, although not necessarily in the therapy room. Being the employee of the therapist may not be necessary, but would further reinforce the subordinate relationship of the supervisee.

On non-Medicare claims, it might be advisable to highlight the possibility that services were performed by either the supervisor or supervisee. Invoices could be printed with the supervisor's name in larger print and listing the supervisees' names. A statement that all services are provided by the supervisor or directly under his or her supervision could be included. A similar rubber stamp might be routinely applied to insurance forms. Given such information, it may not be necessary to have the supervisee sign the claim. It is clear, however, that should the insurance company request further information, the identity of the therapist must be clearly indicated.

DIAGNOSES, IDENTIFIED PATIENTS, AND PROCEDURE CODES

Practitioners should honestly list only those services actually provided. There may be instances, however, when the service or identified patient is not obvious.

Few insurance policies cover marriage counseling or "marital therapy." Most require an individual to be identified, with a "medical" diagnosis, as the focus of treatment. In a marital crisis, it is not unusual for one or both parties to be suffering from significant anxiety or depression, which may be appropriately diagnosed as dysthymic, anxiety, adjustment, or other disorders. Many therapists will identify one member of the couple as the patient, and list both individual and conjoint sessions under that individual's name. It would clearly be unethical to file two insurance claims (one for Mr. Jones and one for Mrs. Jones) for a single therapy session. Whether it is ethical, when one or both parties have legitimate diagnoses, to list only one as a patient in a joint psychotherapy session may be a more subtle question.

Some therapists believe that when one patient is the focus of treatment and both are present, it is acceptable to list the services under that person's name. Others maintain that they are treating two *individuals* in a conjoint session. Clearly those who are "treating the marriage" will find that their conceptual system fits least well into an insurance company's definition of reimbursable service.

Questions of who is the identified patient also arise frequently when dealing with children. Good clinical practice often involves seeing a child alone and with the family, as well as seeing the parent(s) without the child. In any of these contexts, the child legitimately remains the identified patient. Meeting with the parents to aid them in helping their child is appropriate therapy. Questions arise as to which procedure code would be most applicable when the child is not physically present. Some practitioners consider "individual therapy" to be a generic term that applies to individual, family, and other sessions as long as the focus is on the identified patient (see Chapter 3).

Under this same reasoning, hypnosis and biofeedback should not need to be separately listed any more than would guided imagery or behavioral intervention, as long as they are legitimate tools of the therapist's individual treatment. Others believe that it is necessary to specifically differentiate individual therapy, family therapy, and collateral contact.

Although there is some legitimate disagreement about reporting family sessions, misrepresenting group therapy as individual psychotherapy is clearly unacceptable. Group therapy is generally reimbursed at a significantly lower rate per patient than individual therapy. To indicate to an insurance company that eight individuals each received 1 hour of "individual psychotherapy" at the same time would probably be considered fraudulent.

Insurance companies will rarely pay for late cancellations or "no shows." Although it is legitimate to charge a patient for this time, the session should not be listed as "psychotherapy."

Occasionally therapists spend long periods of time on the telephone with a patient during a crisis or because the patient was unable to come into the office. Therapists, like accountants and lawyers, should see their professional time on the telephone to be equally as valuable as face-to-face contact. Unfortunately, insurance companies do not usually consider telephone consultations to be reimbursable. One might be tempted to bill a telephone session as "psychotherapy," because one is providing a service similar to what would be provided in the therapist's office. Although possibly illegal, I know of no situations where therapists have been prosecuted for listing legitimate telephone sessions as *psychotherapy*.

Nevertheless, the more conservative approach would be to list a telephone session as such, and to use the appropriate procedure code (e.g., 90831). Unfortunately, this is likely to lead to denial of the claim or, at best, to a lengthy appeal.

Therapists also question the use of diagnostic codes. Insurance policies usually will pay for most regular *DSM-III-R* and *ICD-9* codes but not for the "V codes," including marital problems, academic problems, or uncomplicated bereavement. Under managed care, some insurance companies are refusing to pay for personality disorders, adjustment disorders, and some other conditions, and are reserving payment only for severe and acute problems.

As discussed in Chapter 3, therapists express concern about listing either "mild" diagnoses, which might result in denial of claims, or "severe" ones, which could have deleterious effects on the patient. It is clearly fraudulent to list a flagrantly incorrect diagnosis. On the other hand, there may be several legitimate choices, and the impact of choosing one diagnosis over another should be carefully considered. For example, an individual may initially present with an adjustment problem but also have a severe personality disorder. If the therapist expects the therapy to be long term, he or she is well advised to list both diagnoses, because the insurance company might question 2 or 3 years of treatment for an adjustment disorder. On the other hand, a patient may come in for treatment of a very focused problem and not want deeper personality exploration. Although the therapist may note a personality disorder, he or she should probably list only the Axis I adjustment disorder. Likewise, a patient who is functioning in a job but is suspected of a schizo-affective disorder might as easily be diagnosed as having a depressive disorder, especially if fellow employees or the employer are likely to become aware of the diagnosis.

CONFIDENTIALITY

Confidentiality is a crucial consideration in mental health practice. Through training, experience, and knowledge of the law, ethical practitioners keep the details of all psychotherapy confidential. Of course, the patient has the right to authorize that the practitioner divulge specific information to specified third parties. The insurer also has a legitimate right to request information to determine whether the patient is eligible for treatment under the terms of the insurance contract. Thus, the insurer may need to know specific services and diagnosis. As a utilization control measure, insurance companies may also require documentation such as summaries or progress notes. In fact, one aspect of managed care is the increasing review of the specific process of therapy, rather than just accepting the therapist's statement that certain services were necessary.

Revealing services rendered, diagnoses, and even progress notes (with the patient's permission) might inconvenience the therapist, but would create few ethical problems if the material remained truly confidential. Surprisingly, there seem to be no laws or regulations requiring third-party payers to keep such information confidential. Although most insurance companies seem to be fairly scrupulous in this regard, an individual therapist can never guarantee confidentiality once information is released to a third party. This would be true even if there were more stringent legal safeguards.

A more common confidentiality problem involves the claims-processing route. Claims frequently must be submitted to the personnel department of the company that employs the patient. Even when these individuals are given training regarding confidentiality, the likelihood of "gossip" spreading is far greater than in the licensed professions. When the claims are processed directly by the insurer, there is still a small possibility that the claim could be handled by an acquaintance of the patient. In fact, I know of several such instances. Confidentiality is a problem that should be addressed not only by mental health therapists, but also by health professionals in general. It is no less important that a vasectomy, venereal disease, or even corns on the feet be kept confidential, than it is to protect a patient's privacy in the treatment of schizophrenia, depression, or a child's conduct disorder.

The Health Insurance Association of America and the American Psychiatric Association ("Reimbursement: A Simple Coding," 1985) sponsored an alternate psychiatric coding system for insurance claims reporting. It uses only six diagnostic categories, which are a synthesis of diagnosis, level of impairment, prognosis, and indications for treatment. Using these categories would significantly help protect confidentiality, but unfortunately would probably not be accepted by insurance companies.

It is important that patients understand the limits of confidentiality. Practitioners should receive written consent (often included on the insurance form) to release information, but also should explain to the patient the possible limits of confidentiality. The therapist should help the patient to weigh the financial advantages of releasing information against possible hazards. Although most of my patients elect to receive their insurance benefits, a few have elected to forego reimbursement in order to insure total privacy.

Once again, it is crucial that therapists understand the nature of the insurance contract and share the implications with their patients. Agreeing to seek reimbursement often also means consenting to give up certain information. Under managed-care systems, agreeing to participate may allow the third party to interfere with treatment through its reimbursement systems.

REIMBURSEMENT AUTHORIZATION VERSUS TREATMENT RESPONSIBILITY

Insurers will generally pay only for treatment that they determine to be "medically necessary and appropriate." Under managed care systems, utilization reviewers often reject approval of payment for requested services. These reviewers are often general nurses or other nonmental health care professionals whose reviews are frequently monitored by mental health professionals.

Insurance companies claim they do not dictate treatment, but merely what will be approved for reimbursement. Given the high cost of health care, it is clear that determining reimbursement strongly influences what care will be provided by the therapist and accepted by the patient. Nevertheless, insurance companies apparently have the right to determine what is reimbursable and it might take an official challenge (through insurance commissions or courts) to make a change.

It is important for practitioners to understand the difference between services authorized (for payment) by an insurance company and the therapist's opinion regarding appropriate treatment. Third parties cannot truly authorize or refuse *treatment*, only *payment*. Professional judgment and ethical concerns often determine the course of treatment, even when an insurance company disagrees. Practitioners are not usually obligated to begin treatment with a patient; however, once treatment has begun, they are mandated by professional ethics and legal considerations to provide appropriate treatment or make an adequate referral.

Wickline v. California (Hogue, 1988a, 1988b; Hotchkiss, 1987) makes these issues salient. Wickline underwent surgery three times for problems associated with her back and legs. After the third operation, her physician wanted her to stay in the hospital 8 days past her scheduled discharge date. Medi-Cal (California's Medicaid) approved only a 4-day extension. None of the physicians appealed the decision, and Wickline was released. She was later readmitted to the hospital and eventually had her right leg amputated. The California Court of Appeals invalidated her suit against Medi-Cal, reasoning that the physicians, and not Medi-Cal were responsible for her discharge.

It is clear that practitioners can be subject to malpractice suits and ethical complaints if they acquiesce to a utilization review determination with which they disagree. It is still not apparent how the courts might view a more rigorous protest of utilization review. For example, the *Wickline* decision has not been tested by the U.S. Supreme Court and therefore does not apply nationwide. It should also be noted that other court decisions have found third party payers conducting utilization review partially responsible for damages after denying payment for treatment (D. Safir, personal communication, December 18, 1990; Hinden, 1988).

Nevertheless, practitioners should always remember that only they can decide on appropriate treatment. At this point, it is prudent to assume that a practitioner has a duty to protest an insurance company decision which he or she sees as harmful. It is also probably the therapist's responsibility to continue treatment until an appropriate referral can be made. Thus practitioner's may be "caught between a rock and a hard place." Insurance companies may refuse to pay for services and the therapist may still be ethically and legally required to provide them. Options include requiring full payment from the patient (if resources are available), making a referral, or seeing the patient on a reduced fee or "gratis" basis (McSweeny, 1987).

CHAPTER 5
FREEDOM OF CHOICE AND MANDATED MENTAL HEALTH

Various state laws have increased the availability of mental health services to citizens. Many large corporations, however, have been able to circumvent the intent of state legislatures through self-insured plans and other loopholes.

FREEDOM OF CHOICE

Freedom of Choice laws, perhaps more accurately called *direct recognition* statutes, require health insurers to recognize specific qualified providers of health care for reimbursement of services covered by insurance policies in that state without the need for referral, billing, or supervision by another profession (Frank, 1982). These state laws may apply to psychologists, social workers, marriage and family therapists, or other defined providers.

Previous to the enactment of such statutes, most insurance policies covered mental health services provided by all physicians, whether it be psychiatrists, family practitioners, or even surgeons. Few policies explicitly recognized psychologists, social workers, or other mental health professionals. Sometimes, physician referrals or physician supervision were required as conditions for reimbursement. Occasionally, insurers would honor independent services by nonphysicians, but this decision was often made at the claims processor or supervisor level, and did not set precedent.

Freedom of Choice laws require that if an insurance policy covers specific mental health services by a physician, it must also cover the same services provided by the other professionals named in the statute. These laws do not mandate coverage for mental health services, nor do they require that the policy cover other nonspecified services provided by psychologists, social workers, or other qualified providers. Furthermore, the laws still reserve certain procedures (e.g., administering ECT or prescribing psychotropic medications) to physicians. If an insurer in a state with a psychologist and social worker Freedom of Choice law covers psychotherapy by psychiatrists, it must also reimburse for psychotherapy by qualified psychologists and social workers. Typically, the insurer is not required to pay for psychological testing or psychosocial histories unless these are also reimbursed for physicians.

New Jersey passed the first direct recognition statute in 1972, recognizing psychologists as providers. As of 1987, approximately 40 states and the District of Columbia had Freedom of Choice statutes recognizing psychologists (Stromberg et al., 1988). By 1989, 15 states plus the District of Columbia recognized social workers (Whiting, 1989), while only California and Florida provided direct recognition for marriage and family therapists ("Practice Issues: Social Workers," 1987).

Practitioners should examine the particular direct recognition statutes in their states to determine criteria for eligibility. The lack of agreement among social workers as to the necessary credentials for independent clinical practice has been a major obstacle to both licensure and direct recognition in many states. Social workers interested in clinical autonomy have fought opposition not only from psychiatrists, psychologists, and insurance companies, but also among themselves. Psychologists have faced the opposition of insurance companies and psychiatrists but have had less dissension from within their own ranks.

Requirements for recognition as a qualified psychologist vary. Most states require insurance companies to reimburse for services of a licensed psychologist. In New Hampshire, in order to receive reimbursement from many carriers, including Blue Cross/Blue Shield, a psychologist must be listed in the National Register of Health Care Providers, a private corporation with more stringent qualifications than those required for state psychology licensure (B. Kanin, personal communication, February 7, 1990). Some states provide Freedom of Choice, but still allow the insurance company to require a physician referral. In Iowa, psychologists must be licensed and also have a Health Service Provider designation, which is similar in stringency to a National Register listing (W. D. McEchron, personal communication, January 22, 1990).

Direct recognition laws do not usually require that therapists from different professions receive equivalent fees. Insurance companies will often reimburse psychiatrists at a higher rate than psychologists, with social workers receiving an even lower reimbursement. Sometimes this fee schedule is implemented by developing UCRs, using each profession as a separate database. At other times, the insurance company arbitrarily allows differential payment for each profession.

EXTRATERRITORIALITY

One major loophole in many Freedom of Choice statutes is *extraterritoriality*. For example, if an individual lives and works in Alabama, a state with psychology Freedom of Choice but no extraterritoriality clause written into the law, and works for a large national company whose contract was written in a different state, the employer is not obligated to honor Alabama's Freedom of Choice legislation, and may decide to exclude reimbursement for psychological services. Many Freedom of Choice laws close the extraterritoriality loophole. State psychological associations report that insurance companies are usually, but not invariably, honoring those provisions.

Most Freedom of Choice laws do not apply to HMOs and PPOs. One exception is Massachusetts, where a mandated benefits law applies Freedom of Choice for psychiatrists, psychologists, licensed independent social workers, and certain nurse practitioners to both insurance and managed-care arrangements, specifically expanding both mandated benefits and direct recognition to HMOs and PPOs (E. Harris, personal communication, January, 1990).

Even in Freedom of Choice states, HMOs and PPOs may exclude psychologists, social workers, and others. These plans are not usually defined as "insurance" and therefore are not usually covered by insurance laws. Also, the mechanism for choosing a panel of providers may, in effect, exclude these professions. For example, an HMO or PPO may allow any member of the active medical staff of a particular hospital to join. If psychologists or social workers are not eligible to be members of the active medical staff, they will also be excluded from the HMO or PPO.

There may be other exceptions to Freedom of Choice. For example, all group plans written in Florida allow Freedom of Choice concerning psychologists. However, individual plans, self-insured trusts, group plans written out of state, and managed-care plans are exempted (Stimel, 1989). Michigan has direct recognition of psychologists for insurance, HMOs, and PPOs. Yet, Blue Cross/Blue Shield of Michigan has devised a way to be virtually exempt from these provisions. Many employers establish contracts with Blue Cross/Blue Shield of Michigan in which all mental health services are to be provided through either *outpatient psychiatric clinics (OPCs)* or physicians. Although OPCs must include psychiatrists, psychologists, and social workers and are subject to various regulations, psychologists and social workers are typically hired under the supervision of psychiatrists who must approve diagnoses and treatment plans. Thus, in practice, Freedom of Choice for Michigan psychologists and social workers has been undermined (R. E. Erard, personal communication, February 13, 1990).

Another obstacle to Freedom of Choice is simple noncompliance. Most refusals to pay valid benefits can be cleared up at the claims processor or supervisor level. However, cases have been reported of outright "stonewalling" by insurance companies. Appeals, even to the state insurance commission, may be necessary to gain full compliance.

ERISA

Probably the most significant threat to Freedom of Choice comes from *ERISA* and self-insured plans. Although Congress passed the Employees Retirement Income Security Act (ERISA) in 1974 to protect the solvency of private pension plans, employers have also used ERISA to evade state insurance laws (Stromberg et al., 1988). In order to protect private pension plans, which were poorly regulated by different state laws, ERISA states "[The] provisions of [ERISA] shall supersede any and all state laws in so far as they may now or hereafter relate to any employee benefit plan [covered by ERISA]" (American Psychological Association, memorandum, October 17, 1985, p. 1).

The insurance industry has never been regulated by the federal government. The 1945 McCarran-Ferguson Act exempted the "business of insurance" from federal law or regulation and "reserved" it for state regulation. Court cases involving ERISA hinge on definitions of insurance as well as the power of ERISA to supersede state laws.

This situation becomes even more complicated because some plans are truly self-insured, while others purchase insurance to protect themselves against heavy losses. Furthermore, insurance companies may administer a self-insured plan without actually insuring it. Controversy also exists as to whether self-insurance programs administered by insurance companies are entitled to the ERISA exemption. In 1985, the Supreme Court ruled in *Metropolitan Life Insurance Company v. Commonwealth of Massachusetts* (1985) that Freedom of Choice legislation applies to ERISA plans that purchase insurance from insurance companies (Stromberg et al., 1988).

In 1987, the Third District Federal Court ruled in *Insurance Board v. Muir* that companies that are truly self-insured, but that have their plans administered by an insurance company, are exempt from state insurance laws under ERISA. They ruled that "insurers were not engaged in the business of insurance while providing administrative services in the process of health benefit claims for an ERISA plan, with the plan assuming all financial risk" (p. 408). Yet federal courts in other jurisdictions have not always ruled similarly (Knapp & VandeCreek, 1990).

At this time, the eventual impact of ERISA and self-insured plans remains questionable. Reports from various state psychological associations reveal that denial of reimbursement to psychologists by self-insured plans is among the most frequent insurance problems encountered by psychologists.

A major illustration of this problem involves General Motors employees ("Practice Issues: Ohio Psychologists," 1986; "Professional Issues: GM," 1985; Wiggins, 1987). In April, 1985, the United Auto Workers and General Motors agreed to eliminate psychologists from direct payment for services. All referrals to psychologists had to made by a physician or osteopath, and all insurance billing had to be done by the referring physician. At that time, a major attempt by psychologists to overcome General Motors' position was unsuccessful.

Interestingly, United Auto Workers contracts at General Motors, Ford, and Chrysler which begin in July, 1991 and January, 1992 will allow independent practicing psychologists, psychiatric social workers, and clinical nurse specialists to provide services to union employees at these companies (Youngstrom, 1991).

Self-insured companies' regulations can be capricious. Hewlett Packard, a self-insured company plan that is exempt from Freedom of Choice statutes, unilaterally decided to exclude EdD psychologists, many of whom are listed in the National Register, but continues to reimburse marriage and family counselors ("Degree v. Training," 1990; "Hewlett-Packard Continues," 1990).

When faced with self-insured plans that refuse to pay a provider, practitioners have several options. They should first check to see if a plan is truly self-insured. This may be accomplished by contacting the employer, or even the state insurance commissioner.

Practitioners or patients may negotiate directly with plan administrators. If a plan recognizes only psychiatrists, then psychologists or social workers might argue that there are no available psychiatrists, or none with the special expertise needed, to handle a specific problem. These negotiations are more likely to succeed if the self-insured plan is relatively small. Nevertheless, if a plan is truly self-insured and refuses to pay, there seems to be little legal recourse.

MANDATED MENTAL HEALTH COVERAGE

By 1989, 27 states had some form of mandated mental health legislation ("Legislation: The Slowdown," 1989). These laws require all insurance contracts to include specific minimal services. They may specify particular mental health services and sometimes establish minimum dollar amounts or numbers of visits. Connecticut requires an insurance company to pay at least 50% for outpatient mental health services with a yearly cap of not less than $2,000 (R.M. Lee, personal communication, November 17, 1990). Psychologists, psychiatrists, clinical nurse specialists, and social workers are eligible.

Maryland (Maryland Psychological Association, 1990) requires all major medical policies to reimburse subscribers for at least 30 days of inpatient treatment and for outpatient expenses required due to "acute mental illnesses and emotional disorders which, in the professional judgment of practitioners, are subject to significant improvement through short term therapy" (p. 20). These services must be reimbursed for at least 65% of the benefit level provided for other types of illnesses for the first 20 visits, and 50% of the benefit level provided for other types of illnesses for the remaining visits. Some states, such as Florida, require that optional coverage be offered for mental and nervous disorders and that such coverage be at the same rate as for physical illness.

More mandated mental health benefits will probably be enacted. In many states there is strong support for laws covering substance abuse, but less enthusiasm for mandating other mental health services.

As with Freedom of Choice, a major peril to such bills comes from ERISA. It appears at this time that Congress may soon consider legislation that would definitively decide whether ERISA preempts mandated benefits legislation for self-insured plans (Stromberg et al., 1988). Such legislation would have momentous effects on the practices of psychologists, social workers, and other practitioners who are affected by their state's Freedom of Choice laws. If National Health Insurance becomes law and is implemented through the private sector, it will probably mandate some minimal level of mental health services.

CHAPTER 6
PRIVATE AND
QUASI-PRIVATE INSURERS

Despite the expansion of government programs and pressures for a national health insurance plan, most Americans find their health coverage provided by private companies or such organizations as Blue Cross/Blue Shield.

BLUE CROSS AND BLUE SHIELD

The concept of providing health care services in exchange for monthly payments reportedly began in Dallas in 1929 when a hospital administrator offered to provide local teachers a maximum of 20 days of hospital care for 50 cents per month. In the 1930s, the popularity of hospital insurance grew nationally. As hospitals offering insurance formed networks, these eventually became Blue Cross/Blue Shield (BC/BS) companies (Pennsylvania Blue Shield, 1989a). Although traditional BC/BS plans may be diminishing, in 1987 they still provided hospitalization insurance to approximately one-third of Americans, and coverage of physician services to approximately one-quarter. In many local areas, BC/BS covers a majority of policy holders (Stromberg et al., 1988).

The administrative structure of BC/BS can be complex. Each Blue Cross and each Blue Shield is a separate, state-chartered, nonprofit organization. Several separate corporations may cover a state. For example, Pennsylvania has four separate regional Blue Cross organizations and one statewide Blue Shield.

Although they are nonprofit companies, supposedly organized for the benefit of the citizens, BC/BS plans have been traditionally more responsive to the needs of hospitals and physician providers than to the public. Furthermore, as the professional boards were dominated by individuals in more established professions (primarily MDs, DDSs, and DMDs), they have resisted expanding benefits to other health care professions such as psychologists, optometrists, and nurse practitioners. Nevertheless, this is changing due to public, professional, and legislative pressures, and as more lay members and other professionals are wielding influence on BC/BS boards.

Blue Cross generally covers hospital expenses. These include room costs and the charges for services provided by the hospital. Blue Shield pays for the services of physicians and other providers.

Occasionally, Blue Cross may cover a mental health practitioner's costs. This occurs if the hospital bills Blue Cross directly for services and then pays the practitioner. The hospital may include the cost of mental health services in the *per diem* (daily rate) or charge separately for these services. The practitioner may be a salaried employee or one paid by the hospital on a fee-for-service basis.

Hospital services provided by most private practitioners will be reimbursed through Blue Shield. A participating practitioner will bill Blue Shield and be paid directly by them. A nonparticipating therapist may file with Blue Shield or let the patient do so. Blue Shield will pay the patient when a practitioner is nonparticipating.

Many Blue Shield plans do not cover outpatient psychotherapy. These services are often reimbursed through a *major medical plan*, which may be part of BC/BS or purchased separately from another company. Reimbursement for outpatient psychotherapy is often more limited than for the same inpatient services. Whether outpatient therapy is covered under Blue Shield varies not only from state to state, but also among the different plans offered to different employers by the same Blue Shield.

BC/BS pioneered the concept of *participating providers*. To participate, practitioners agree to accept Blue Shield's determination as full payment for their services. In exchange, Blue Shield pays them directly, thus guaranteeing payment. The disadvantage is that payments are likely to be lower (and never higher) than what practitioners would otherwise charge.

Blue Shield plans have typically been based on *usual, customary, and reasonable (UCR)* charges. As explained in Chapter 2, this means that Blue Shield will pay either the practitioner's usual charge for a service, or the customary fee for the area, whichever is lower. Although they will pay a "reasonable" charge for an unusual clinical circumstance, this occurs very rarely. UCRs are calculated within professions. In a particular geographical area, the customary psychotherapy charge for psychiatrists, psychologists, and social workers might be very different. The charges allowed in one geographical area might also differ significantly from allowed charges in other locales.

Under UCRs, payment schedules lag by at least a year. For example, a psychiatrist might raise her fee in September, 1991, from $105 to $110. In September, 1992, her fee might increase to $115. If Blue Shield bases its UCR for July 1, 1992 to June 30, 1993 on her 1991 usual charges, she might still be receiving $105, when her actual fee has risen to $115. Furthermore, many plans are "freezing" fees, limiting increases to less than inflation, or revising fee schedules less often than annually. These strategies keep UCRs well below true prevailing rates.

By agreeing to participate, one *must* accept the Blue Shield allowance as full payment and may not bill the patient for more than the allowed fee. If there is a co-payment in the contract, the therapist collects the co-payment from the patient but still must accept Blue Shield's determination of the total allowable charge.

Many Blue Shield programs have special low-income plans. The Blue Shield reimbursement, which must be accepted by participating providers as full payment, will often be substantially lower (often 50% or less) than for those individuals under a UCR plan. In some states, it is the practitioner's responsibility to ascertain whether a patient meets the income eligibility requirements for a patient who is in such a plan.

Deciding whether to participate in Blue Shield depends on each practitioner's situation. For therapists in states without a Freedom of Choice law for their profession, participation may not be an option. Furthermore, even in some states with Freedom of Choice, participating providership has not been offered to psychologists or social workers.

Mental health professionals with substantial hospital practices may find it advantageous to be Blue Shield participating providers. This is particularly true for those performing consultations, or treating hospital patients who may not continue as office patients. Patients seen only in consultation often have little understanding as to why the consultation was ordered, and later may resent receiving a bill. If a practitioner is a nonparticipating provider, Blue Shield will pay the patient, who may keep the reimbursement rather than paying the provider. Even patients who pay the provider often do not feel obligated to pay the difference between the provider's charges and the Blue Shield allowance. Patients in the hospital often feel that Blue Shield's allowance is the "reasonable" charge and that anything in excess is unreasonable "gouging."

Therapists with limited hospital practices are less likely to be participating providers. For practitioners who treat only their own regular patients in the hospital, full payment does not tend to be as much of a problem, because of the ongoing relationship.

If Blue Shield covers a substantial number of outpatients in a therapist's practice, the decision on whether to participate becomes somewhat more difficult, analogous to that of participating in various managed-care plans. If the Blue Shield UCR is close to the provider's usual charge, the practitioner may find it worthwhile to participate. This may attract patients who will have small co-payments. Participation may reduce paperwork for the therapist and simplify billing. On the other hand, by participating, a therapist who generally collects payment at each session would face some inconvenience as well as some collection delays.

Some Blue Shield plans have special "quirks." For example, several major Blue Shield companies do not pay for psychological testing in most or all of their plans, even if the patient is in the hospital (see Chapter 3, p. 23). Although they provide a procedure code for this service, using that code will invariably prompt a computerized response noting that the particular subscriber's plan does not cover that service. Blue Shield will claim a willingness to include testing in their plans but say that the employer/subscriber has not requested the inclusion of psychological testing. It is difficult to believe that each employer who negotiates a contract specifically considers and rejects psychological testing. More likely, a prototype plan is offered. Few employers would think to look up psychological testing specifically and ask for its inclusion. If they did, Blue Shield would include it in their plan at an increased premium.

Therapists should be aware of some reimbursement limitations with Blue Shield and other insurers. Blue Shield will sometimes refuse to reimburse common and well-accepted clinical practices. For instance, family therapy has been an acceptable part of clinical practice for over 25 years, yet some Blue Shield plans will reject a claim using a family therapy code. Similarly, biofeedback is often rejected. Responsible professional care in the hospital may include psychotherapy by the patient's outpatient nonphysician therapist with medical management by a physician or psychiatrist. As discussed in Chapter 3, if the two practitioners use similar codes, Blue Shield will usually reject one, claiming that only one unit of service can be given in a day. Practitioners in hospitals need to coordinate their services and coding, so that legitimate descriptions are given, but also so that both individuals will be paid.

Each Blue Shield company tends to have its own idiosyncrasies. For example, Montana plans do not typically pay for psychological evaluations unless referred by a medical doctor or performed in a medical setting (J. Maeder, personal communication, February 13, 1990). Practitioners in some states have reported good relationships and acceptable treatment by Blue Shield. For example, Blue Shield covers psychological testing and pays what many psychologists consider to be a fairly reasonable charge in Massachusetts. However, Massachusetts offers no option for a practitioner to be a nonparticipating provider and still see Blue Shield patients (E. Harris, personal communication, February, 1990). The psychologist UCR in Michigan is quite low, based on 75% of the "out state" rate for psychiatrists. Most Michigan psychologists decline becoming participating providers (R. E. Erard, personal communication, February 13, 1990). Furthermore, as mentioned earlier, BC/BS of Michigan has evaded Freedom of Choice regulations through a complex system of outpatient psychiatric clinics. New Hampshire BC/BS requires psychologists to be listed in the National Register of Health Care Providers (B. Kanin, personal communication, February 7, 1990). Alabama psychologists report few problems with BC/BS (R. Meredith, personal communication, January, 1990).

Historically, BC/BS plans have presented themselves as "provider plans" with supposedly more humanistic policies than the more mercenary commercial insurers; as fee-based payers; and as the insurer of last resort for people who could not obtain commercial insurance (Stromberg et al., 1988). In response to commercial insurers' taking the lowest risk patients, the increasing costs of health care, and public and legislative pressure, BC/BS plans have now instituted cost controls and utilization review as well as many other limitations. They have also developed managed-care concepts. Although differences between BC/BS and commercial plans are rapidly fading, BC/BS plans will probably continue to play an important role as major third-party payers in the future.

COMMERCIAL INSURERS

As difficult as it is to make broad statements about BC/BS programs, it is impossible to generalize about other private insurers. As many as two-thirds of people not in government programs may have their health insurance covered by AETNA, Metropolitan, Prudential, Travelers, CIGNA, Equitable, and other commercial companies. Traditionally, commercial insurers concentrated on hospital services, paying less attention to physician and other provider services (Stromberg et al., 1988). Virtually all patients covered by commercial plans will be part of a group, usually from their employment. Individual coverage from commercial insurers is either not available, or much more expensive, than BC/BS coverage.

The Consolidated Omnibus Budget Reconciliation Act (COBRA) was enacted by the U.S. Congress in 1985. COBRA provides options for continued group insurance coverage for a limited period of time to employees who have lost group insurance benefits because of job termination or reduced work hours (U.S. Department of Labor, 1990). After terminating a job, individuals are usually allowed 1 to 3 months' extended coverage at the group rate. Some states require private insurers to provide coverage to individuals for a specified period (usually 6 to 18 months) after termination of employment at an individual rate. Commercial insurers sometimes allow indefinite extension, but at the expensive individual rates.

Typically, commercial plans exclude services not ordered by a "doctor," injuries due to war, preexisting conditions, and other circumstances. As previously discussed, limitations on preexisting conditions can create obvious problems. Usually insurers will not pay for these for at least a year. An individual might have had several panic attacks as an adolescent, remained symptom-free for many years, and developed anxiety symptoms in his forties. He could easily claim that this is a "new illness" rather than a "preexisting condition." Other situations may be more problematic. An individual with recurring depressive episodes, who had functioned fairly well for 2 years, might have a major depressive episode. Is this considered a preexisting condition? Most insurance companies ask when the symptom or illness first appeared and when the therapist was first consulted. The answers to these questions might be used to define a preexisting condition. Other insurance companies define a preexisting condition as one for which medical treatment was sought in some designated period of time. Therapists should be aware of the reimbursement implications of their answers, but also the need to not give inaccurate information to the insurer.

Commercial insurers will generally pay only for treatment that they determine to be "medically necessary" and appropriate. Equitable Insurance requires "medical necessity" and an MD or PhD, unless otherwise ordered by law. Psychologists review psychological cases, while psychiatrists review psychiatric cases. They require a *DSM-III-R* diagnosis. In psychologists' cases, the patient and psychologist participate in completing the review forms. For psychiatrists' patients, only the psychiatrist completes the form. Treatment progress must be shown and must coordinate with professional understanding of the case and how this relates to the results. Treatment progress or reasons for a lack of progress must be shown (K. Berc, personal communication, February 27, 1990).

Although insurance plans differ greatly, some features are typical. Under most plans, inpatient mental health services are reimbursed at between 80% and 100% of customary fees. Commercial insurers usually pay for psychological testing, psychotherapy, and psychiatric/psychological consultations. Most companies do not seem to have individual provider profiles but have limits based on customary fees in a geographical area. Typically, no more than 30 inpatient days are allowed per hospitalization, and there is often a yearly limit, such as 90 days.

Coverage for outpatient psychotherapy is usually much more limited than for inpatient treatment. Patient co-payments may range from 0% to 50%. This is often combined with a maximum allowable fee, sometimes as low as $25. Thus, a plan might pay 50% of outpatient mental health fees, up to an "allowable" charge of $40. In reality, this plan would pay a maximum of $20 per session. A therapist whose fee is $100 would thus receive $20 reimbursement for each session. This therapist would be permitted (and probably obligated) to collect the remaining $80 from the patient.

Many private plans allow assignment. Practitioners who accept assignment are generally under no obligation to accept the allowed charge as a full fee and may bill the entire balance. It is my experience that, even when the patients do not sign for assignment and have paid in full, insurance companies still often send payment to the practitioner.

In addition to per-session limits, many private insurers have annual deductibles, usually between $100 and $1,000. These may apply to an entire family or to each family member. As health care costs increase, deductibles and patient co-payments are likely to rise. Higher deductibles preserve the important concept that insurance should cover more devastating losses. A more insidious tendency is to limit mental health costs. Because many plans have "caps" as low as $500 per year, the first five or six visits may be well covered, but there is no reimbursement beyond those sessions. For an individual or family in severe crisis or with a serious mental illness, this type of coverage leaves them highly vulnerable to catastrophic losses. Insurance companies may also limit the number of outpatient sessions per year.

Many private carriers respond to claims with excellent statements that indicate the amount charged, amount allowed, deductibles, co-payments, and the insurance company's actual payment. They often have computer-generated explanations of the rationale for reduced payments. These allow the practitioner or patient to assess quickly whether an error has occurred. Other companies merely send a statement with the date of service and amount of payment, sometimes even omitting the date of service. This response leaves both the practitioner and subscriber baffled as to the reasoning behind the particular reimbursement.

It is important to realize how often errors are made. Occasionally, these are due to flaws in the master computer programs, but most often they are the result of clerical mistakes by the claims processor. Of course, the error may also have occurred in the practitioner's office. Many therapists suspect a pattern of "intentional mistakes" by insurance companies.

I would estimate that at least 20% of the claims filed by our office are processed incorrectly. Rarely is the error to the advantage of the practitioner or patient. The most frequent mistakes are reimbursement of inpatient services as if they were outpatient and incorrect procedure codes. Recently, a psychotherapy claim was denied with the explanation that "routine health care physicals" are not part of the coverage.

A follow-up letter usually corrects the problem, although there is sometimes unwarranted delay. If there is any doubt concerning the reimbursement, it is usually advisable to write a letter of inquiry indicating the reimbursement one would expect. It helps, too, if the practitioner can "second guess" the insurance company, trying to figure out which codes they might have used and correcting the apparent error. Including copies of the initial claim and any notices received from the insurance company also expedites correction.

Providers report varying experiences with commercial carriers. The major companies seem to process claims and respond to appeals fairly quickly. Yet a number of practitioners have reported disputes with insurance companies that have lasted for several years, including many letters which are long ignored. Consider writing your state's Insurance Commissioner when claims or letters are ignored. Insurance Commissioners can provide complaint guidelines and forms.

SELF-INSURED TRUSTS

As discussed earlier, self-insured trusts are usually exempt from Freedom of Choice or mandated mental health insurance laws. Self-insured trusts may be established by a company or a union. They are often administered by insurance companies, health care administration companies, the employer, unions, or even by local banks. Self-insured trusts are not truly "insurance." Instead, a company or union decides to forego health insurance and take the financial risk itself. Sometimes companies will provide most of the health benefits from their own revenue but buy insurance to protect themselves against especially high losses.

Mental health coverage under these plans varies widely. Some require mental health care to be provided by psychiatrists, while others may allow psychologists with PhDs, all licensed psychologists, or any type of therapist that the specific plan allows. Coverage ranges from 0% to 100%. Deductibles, caps, and per-visit maximums may exist.

The variety of health plans and differing coverage reinforces the advisability of being knowledgeable about the coverage available in all of the major plans in your locale. It also underscores the importance of not relying on patients' impressions of their coverage and reiterating to all patients that they are ultimately responsible for payment regardless of coverage or reimbursement.

CHAPTER 7
GOVERNMENT PROGRAMS

Prior to 1965, very little health care was covered by government programs. Medicare, Medicaid, CHAMPUS, and other government programs are now major third-party reimbursers and appear to be setting trends for future health care coverage.

MEDICARE

Medicare and Medicaid legislation were established in 1965 as a component of President Lyndon Johnson's "Great Society." These programs reflected an evolution of attitudes, which began with President Franklin Roosevelt's New Deal, about federal responsibility for health care benefits. During World War II, when many Americans had health care provided by the government, this trend accelerated. After the war, many people continued to expect benefits through the Veterans Administration or other governmental entities. By the 1960s, concern about the cost of health care led to Medicare and Medicaid being established to provide for the elderly and for children of indigent parents (Wright, 1990).

Developments in Medicare are crucial to all mental health practitioners, not only because this program serves such a large population, but also because other carriers use Medicare as a prototype. Federal, state, and private plans often excerpt language from Medicare statutes to apply to other plans. Medicare is likely to be the model for any future national health insurance.

Organized medicine initially strongly opposed Medicare as the first step toward "socialized medicine." To win acceptance, the legislation was based on a "fee-for-service" model and utilized a UCR concept. The latter was a key factor in the increasing cost of all health care since 1965.

Medicare currently insures 30 million individuals, mostly 65 or older, who are eligible for other Social Security benefits. In addition, it also pays for health care of people who are considered disabled under the stringent Social Security requirements.

Medicare is administered by the Health Care Financing Administration (HCFA) of the Department of Health and Human Services (HHS). HCFA contracts with insurance companies to process and pay Medicare claims. These organizations, called *fiscal intermediaries* under Part A and *carriers* under Part B, determine reasonable charges and conduct audits for a geographical area. Thus, HHS and Congress create the broadest general policy. HCFA makes national decisions on categories of reimbursement, while the local intermediary makes more limited decisions about specific coverage and reimbursement (American Psychological Association, undated-a; Stromberg et al., 1988).

Medicare Part A is an "entitlement" program available to all eligible individuals and does not require a premium. Part A covers inpatient care, hospital or skilled nursing facilities, and some home care. Services of a mental health practitioner are generally not included under Part A. If a mental health practitioner's services are included in a hospital's per diem rate, these services could be eligible under Part A; however, this exception does not usually apply for therapists in private practice.

Part B, also called "Supplementary Medical Insurance," is an optional service and involves the patient's paying a monthly premium. Most Part A enrollees also subscribe to Part B (Stromberg et al., 1988).

Until recently, only physicians were eligible for reimbursement for psychotherapy under Medicare Part B. Psychologists could obtain reimbursement only for psychological testing, and only if referred by a physician. No other mental health practitioners were eligible for reimbursement.

In 1989, Congress passed a bill requiring Medicare to reimburse both psychologists and social workers for outpatient services. These professionals are required to notify the patient's primary physician after treatment has begun, unless the patient specifically requests that no notice be given. This law went into effect on July 1, 1990.

Although HCFA had more than 6 months to work on implementation, when the law went into effect they had not even written temporary regulations. Thus, many Medicare carriers continued to deny claims for many months after psychologists and social workers were legally eligible. The immense confusion among professionals and the inconvenience to patients may be a typical result of both bureaucratic sluggishness and counterlobbying by those opposed to the legislation. It also illustrates the fact that legislative gains need to be carefully monitored with special attention to the language and implementation of guidelines.

When HCFA finally issued regulations, it indicated that only psychologists with a PhD in *Clinical Psychology* and certain social workers would be eligible for reimbursement. Further, they indicated that psychologists and social workers could not independently bill for inpatient psychotherapy. Their services could be billed only under Part A, as part of the DRG allotment. Thus, a hospital using psychologists or social workers would receive the same amount as one not using them, creating a disincentive to use their services. Psychiatrists could continue to bill independently, under Part B, for hospital psychotherapy.

To rectify what seemed like HCFA's disregard for the intent of the previous legislation, Congress passed a "technical amendment" mandating that psychologists and social workers be allowed to bill directly for inpatient services.

As of February, 1991, permanent HCFA regulations still had not been written. HCFA had verbally agreed to expand the definition of *eligible clinical psychologist* to include PsyDs and perhaps EdDs from programs which are clinical in nature, although perhaps not using that title. It was less likely that licensed clinical psychologists with Masters degrees would be eligible for reimbursement.

Another aspect of the legislation was the requirement that psychologists and social workers consult with the patient's primary physician. Although final guidelines have not been written, it appears that when they apply for a Medicare provider number, psychologists and social workers will have to sign an "attestation agreement" that they will consult with "the patient's attending or primary care physician in accordance with accepted professional ethical norms, taking into consideration patient confidentiality" (personal communication, B. Welch, October 30, 1990).

Medicare has devised a tortuous way of computing benefits so that Medicare pays 50% of the approved amount. Reimbursement is limited to 62.5% of "the allowable charge" for services provided for a psychiatric diagnosis to a noninpatient beneficiary, regardless of the "physician's specialty" (Pennsylvania Blue Shield, 1990-1991).

> The 62.5% outpatient psychiatric limitation is calculated as follows:
>
> - The reasonable charge is determined;
> - The reasonable charge is multiplied by .625;
> - Any unsatisfied amount is subtracted; and
> - The balance is multiplied by .80 for payment.
>
> Any mandated reductions (e.g., Gramm-Rudman-Hollings reduction) are withheld after the .80 calculation. (Pennsylvania Blue Shield, 1990-1991, p. 22)

In a typical example, a psychologist might bill $100 per hour for psychotherapy. If Medicare "approved" a $65 charge, they "consider 62.5 percent of allowed psychiatric charges," which is $40.63 (Pennsylvania Blue Shield, Explanation of Benefits Form, 1990). They reimburse 80% of that charge, for a total of $32.50 (or 50% of the approved $65 with a 50% [$32.50] co-payment). Unfortunately, some Medicare carriers are reporting the $40.63 as the "amount approved" and thus misleading the patient into believing that the co-payment is only $8.13. Furthermore, when reported in this fashion, many Medigap policies reimburse only $8.13 rather than the full $32.50.

Until several years ago, Medicare paid 50% of outpatient psychotherapy services, with a maximum yearly reimbursement of $250. This made private psychiatric services unaffordable for many Medicare enrollees. By 1989, the cap was increased to $1,375. As of July, 1990, there is no annual dollar limit for Part B mental health services. All mental health benefits, whether provided by psychiatrists, psychologists, or social workers, will be subject to a 50% co-payment (calculated as shown in the above example) but with no annual limits. Psychological testing, like most nonmental health medical services, requires only a 20% patient co-payment and also has no maximum.

Medicare patients also have a yearly deductible. Many people have "Medigap" insurance which pays both the deductible and co-payments. Most Medigap policies reimburse only for procedures that Medicare has already accepted and reimbursed. As previously mentioned, Medigap may pay the full co-payment or approximately one-quarter of that amount (depending on the Explanation of Benefits form used by the carrier).

Over the past 5 years, Medicare has made many attempts at cost containment. Diagnosis Related Groups (DRGs) have been a main thrust of reducing Part A hospital costs. Under the DRG concept, the hospital is paid a set amount for a particular diagnosis or procedure (e.g., appendectomy) based on the average length of stay and utilization of hospital services for that condition or procedure. It is to the hospital's financial advantage to keep a patient for a shorter period of time because the hospital will receive the same reimbursement regardless of the length of stay. The DRG concept has also been used, more controversially, with mental health units. As of 1988, virtually all freestanding psychiatric hospitals and more than two-thirds of psychiatric units in general hospitals were exempt from DRGs. Inpatients treated on nonpsychiatric units were not exempt (Kiesler & Morton, 1988). Although many medical stays can be predicted with a margin of error of only 1 or 2 days, it is difficult to predict, with any reliability, a typical adequate treatment stay based on a diagnosis such as *depression* or *schizophrenia*.

Cost containment for Part B services has included an increased emphasis on provider participation. Five years ago, a provider was free to choose whether or not to participate in Medicare. By participating and accepting assignment, the practitioner was guaranteed direct payment but was required to accept Medicare's fee. Many providers who charged significantly more than the accepted fee chose not to participate and instead required payment of their full fee directly from the patient. The patient would then receive the allowed charge as partial reimbursement from Medicare.

Several years ago, Medicare encouraged providers to participate by reimbursing more for the services of participating providers than for nonparticipating ones. Furthermore, Medicare published the names of participating providers to encourage patients to patronize them. As of October, 1990, all providers, whether participating or not, are required to file insurance forms for Medicare patients.

Recently Medicare has considered a more heavy-handed effort to increase participation through a concept known as "mandatory assignment." Mandatory assignment requires that practitioners (nonparticipating as well as participating) accept the Medicare prescribed rate (plus the beneficiary's co-payment) as payment in full and not look to the beneficiary or other sources to collect more. Medicare requires mandatory assignment for psychologists and social workers. Psychiatrists still have the option of not participating and collecting their full fee.

Several states, including Pennsylvania, have passed laws prohibiting "balance billing" (Laws of Pennsylvania, Act 1990-81, 1990; "Seniors Like," 1990). These laws require all health care providers to accept fees set by Medicare as payment in full for any patient eligible for Medicare. There is some dispute about whether these laws apply to only those patients using Medicare or to any who are eligible (S. Knapp, personal communication, August, 1990). If the former is true, it will be illegal in states with "balance billing" laws for a therapist to see a Medicare patient at the therapist's regular fee, no matter how low the Medicare reimbursement is or how willing and able the patient is to pay the regular fee. These laws are likely to be tested in the courts.

The amount of Medicare reimbursement varies by region and locality. In other federal programs, reimbursement for psychologists is often 80% of the reimbursement for psychiatrists. Reimbursement for social workers is often 75% of psychiatrists' reimbursement. These same reimbursement formulas have been recommended in the temporary regulations for the 1989 law.

Medicare has also contained costs in the past 5 years by limiting UCR raises. For some years, provider payment rates were "frozen." At other times, they were allowed to rise only by a specific percentage, often below the inflation rate. Sometimes a certain percentage was withheld (e.g., for parts of 1989-1990, all claims were automatically reduced by 2.092%).

In 1991, Congress did not allocate sufficient funds to pay for Medicare. HCFA suggested that carriers deal with this shortfall by drastically increasing claims processing time (B. J. Gagel, personal communication, January 8, 1991). Pennsylvania Blue Shield responded by increasing their average claims processing from 8 to 60 days (R. E. Johnson, personal communication, January 18, 1991).

Beginning in 1992, Medicare will begin phasing in a uniform, national physician fee schedule to replace payments by "reasonable charge" ("New Medicare Fee," 1989). The system is designed to reward providers who rely more on their knowledge, skill, and time spent with patients, rather than rewarding the use of expensive, high-technology medicine. The effect on mental health services is still unknown.

Medicare has set guidelines concerning services of assistants and supervisees. When the supervising provider is "actively involved in and professionally responsible for" the patient's care, the supervisor's name, *not* the therapist's, should be listed. This is discussed in detail in Chapter 4.

When psychological testing is provided, Medicare has explicitly directed that the specific tests *not* be listed. Reimbursement is per hour, not per test. Although in our office we underline and highlight the number of hours, almost inevitably, the claims are paid as if psychological testing were for only 1 hour. All attempts at noting the actual length of testing seem to be ignored by claims processors. Our form letter was illustrated in Chapter 3, Figure 6, page 32. Although we have never received a letter of apology or any other acknowledgement from the Medicare intermediary, we typically receive another check for the correct additional amount within 3 weeks.

Medicare can be expected to add more bureaucratic mandates at the same time it is limiting payments. In 1990, they required all providers, whether or not participating, to file claims for patients. In 1991, they began requiring providers to list the Unique Physician Identification Number (UPIN) of referring providers.

MEDICAID

Medicaid is a joint federal and state program, enacted in 1965 as Title XIX of the Social Security Act, to pay medical bills for certain low-income individuals. Unlike Medicare, which is entirely financed and regulated by the federal government, Medicaid is a collection of 53 separate state and territorial programs with some overriding consistencies but many different objectives, target populations, and packages of services. Although the federal government determines basic requirements and provides options, each state and territory has its own version of Medicaid (Koyanagi, 1988).

Medicaid operates as a "vendor program" with payments made directly to the provider rather than to eligible individuals. Although co-payments are occasionally required, participating providers must usually accept Medicaid reimbursement as payment in full.

The federal government requires that Medicaid provide: (a) inpatient hospital services (except for mental disorders); (b) outpatient hospital services; (c) physician services (MD or DO); (d) laboratory and x-ray services; (e) skilled nursing facility services (other than care in an institution for mental diseases); (f) early periodic screening, diagnosis, and treatment services for children; (g) family planning services; and (h) nurse midwife services.

At their option, states may render: (a) services provided by professionals who are licensed as practitioners under state law (including psychologists, psychiatric social workers, and other mental health professionals); (b) home health care (which can include mental health services if provided by a home health agency that meets Medicare requirements, or if furnished under the supervision of a registered nurse and prescribed by a physician); (c) clinic services furnished by or under direction of a physician, without regard to whether the clinic itself is administered by a physician; (d) other diagnostic, screening, preventive, and rehabilitation services; (e) psychiatric inpatient hospital services and nursing facility services for individuals aged 65 and over in an institution for mental diseases; (f) intermediate care facility services for persons with mental retardation; (g) inpatient psychiatric hospital services for individuals under the age of 22; (h) any other medical care and any other type of remedial care recognized under state law; (i) targeted case management; and (j) a variety of other services such as dentistry and physical therapy.

Medicaid laws are extremely complex and unwieldy. Various regulations often discourage eligible practitioners from providing services. Frequently, regulations are written by several federal and state agencies, and they sometimes contradict each other. Furthermore, the required paperwork can be very difficult and time-consuming.

As of 1988, 29 states include psychologists in Medicaid and authorize direct reimbursement for services without any requirements for physician supervision. Although supervision is not required, many of the states require physician referral for treatment by a psychologist. Eleven states cover psychiatric social workers.

Federal law allows physician services to be delivered in an office, the patient's home, hospital, nursing facility, or other setting. Most states cover physician services without restriction. A few limit all physician visits (ranging from 12 to 48 visits per year). Others may set limits which vary depending upon service setting.

Many states have the same benefit policies for psychiatrists' services as for other physicians. About 20 states have more restrictive limits for visits to a psychiatrist. Limitations can include restrictions on the number of visits per year (from 1 to 45 or more), maximum dollar reimbursements (e.g., $500 per year), or constraints on covered services. Some states limit services by psychologists or social workers more than services by psychiatrists. Others specifically define the types of services (e.g., psychological testing) that these professionals can perform (Koyanagi, 1988).

The major impediment for independent practitioners in providing mental health services to Medicaid recipients is low reimbursement. Reimbursement is typically far below usual rates and is sometimes as low as 25% of typical fees. In 1989, most Medicaid rates for mental health services ranged from $25 to $50 per hour. Even many community mental health centers receive significantly less than their actual cost of service when they treat Medicaid patients and have to make up the difference from local funds or other subsidies.

Unfortunately, Medicaid provides little incentive for ethical practitioners who want to give their patients maximum therapeutic service. Paperwork and other requirements are more onerous than for any other program and the rate of reimbursement is much less.

Some unethical practitioners have committed grossly fraudulent practices such as billing for patients never seen, sessions that never occurred, and grossly overstating services. For example, practitioners have been known to see a group of patients for short medication reviews and bill Medicaid as if each patient had 1 hour of service. This abuse, plus burgeoning health care costs, has made government regulators and policy makers wary of increasing Medicaid reimbursement.

Medicaid has recently stepped up its antifraud prosecution. In addition to uncovering some genuinely unethical practices, they may also be pursuing ethical mental health professionals in an overly aggressive fashion (Buie, 1989b). In one case, an undercover agent posed as a patient of a psychiatrist and wore a concealed recording device. The agent deliberately contrived to prematurely leave a session that had been scheduled for an hour. The psychiatrist was indicted for wrongly billing New York State $90 for a full session, rather than a shorter one (Moran, 1990).

It should also be noted that a number of other practices are considered fraudulent under Medicare/Medicaid amendments. Individuals may not knowingly or willingly solicit or receive, or offer to pay, any remuneration (including "kickbacks," bribes, or rebates), directly or indirectly, overtly or covertly, in cash or in any other form, in return for purchasing, leasing, ordering, arranging for, or recommending purchase or lease, of any Medicare (or Medicaid) covered good or service or in return for referring anyone to a provider for such a good or service. The only exceptions are payments that constitute *bona fide* volume discounts or price reductions if "properly disclosed" and "appropriately" reflected in the claim. Also excepted are payments to employees, such as commissions paid to salesmen (Stromberg et al., 1988).

Many practices could be considered "kickbacks." Stromberg et al. (1988) includes: (a) arrangements in which practitioners refer "overflow" patients to colleagues with whom they share office space, in return for proportionally reduced share of rent; (b) leases in which the rent is a percentage of gross revenues from the practice and not a fixed amount; (c) routine waivers of co-payments or deductibles as an inducement for patients to use the services of that practitioner; (d) discounts or free goods, such as a scoring service offering a psychologist 1 free assessment for every 10 ordered (i.e., 11 for the price of 10); and (e) joint ventures in which two practitioners (perhaps with different specialties) share revenue based on the number of patients referred from one or the other.

CHAMPUS/CHAMPVA

The Civilian Health and Medical Program of the Uniformed Services (CHAMPUS) serves the families of active and retired military. CHAMPVA is a health benefit for the families of veterans with 100% service-connected disabilities, or the surviving spouse or children of a veteran who dies from a service-connected disability. Generally, the same benefit rules apply for CHAMPUS and CHAMPVA, and the same claims processors handle both CHAMPUS and CHAMPVA claims (Office of Civilian and Medical Program of the Uniformed Services - CHAMPUS, 1988).

CHAMPUS covers more that eight and a half million people and is the largest single health insurance plan in the United States. The original intention was to provide benefits at least as generous as those provided by the most comprehensive plan available to federal employees. Like other health plans, CHAMPUS has contained costs in recent years by excluding certain services and instituting more stringent utilization reviews.

CHAMPUS pioneered Freedom of Choice by making more professions eligible for reimbursement than most government or private programs. In addition to psychiatrists, CHAMPUS includes clinical psychologists who are listed in the National Register of Health Service Providers in Psychology or have equivalent credentials. To be eligible to participate in CHAMPUS, clinical social workers must be licensed or certified in a state offering such certification or by a national organization, have a master's degree, and have at least 2 years or 3,000 hours of post-master's-degree clinical social work practice under the supervision of a master's level social worker in an accredited hospital, mental health center, or other appropriate clinical setting.

Psychiatric nurse specialists are also eligible to provide covered services independent of physician referral and supervision. They must be licensed registered nurses with at least a master's degree in nursing with specialization in psychiatric and mental health nursing, and at least 2 years post-master's degree practice in the field of psychiatric and mental health nursing (including an average of 8 hours of patient contact per week). Alternatively, they can be listed in a CHAMPUS-recognized professionally sanctioned listing of clinical specialists in psychiatric and mental health nursing.

Marriage, family, and pastoral counselors with a master's degree in an appropriate behavioral science field or mental health discipline, and who meet various standards of supervision and experience, may receive reimbursement only if patients are referred by physicians who "coordinate" the treatment. Yet only "psychotherapy" and not "marriage or family counseling" is covered.

Mental health counselors with a master's degree in mental health counseling or an allied health field from a regionally accredited institution and who hold a state license, certificate, or certification by the National Academy of Certified Clinical Mental Health Counselors may see CHAMPUS patients under physician referral and supervision. The physician must actually see the patient, perform an evaluation, and arrive at an initial diagnostic impression prior to the referral. The physician must also provide "oversight" and "supervision" of the treatment (CHAMPUS, 1988).

CHAMPUS specifically excludes certain procedures, but is less restrictive than many programs. For example, "family or conjoint therapy" is reimbursed. In fact, CHAMPUS specifically states that family therapy is a necessary part of hospital treatment of children and adolescents. Interestingly, I have seen no discussions on the clinical differences between "family therapy" (a covered service) and "family counseling" (an excluded service) especially in relation to insurance and "medical" versus "nonmedical" services. Psychoanalysis is included but is subject to a specific review for medical or psychological appropriateness. CHAMPUS includes psychological testing, but unlike Medicare, requires that the specific tests be listed. CHAMPUS explicitly excludes such treatments as transcendental meditation, rolfing, guided imagery, and narcotherapy with LSD.

Outpatient therapy is generally limited to two sessions per week, but these restrictions can be modified upon review. CHAMPUS has a peer review system and generally requires a CHAMPUS Treatment Report every 23 sessions. The report includes questions concerning the progress of the patient, description of the problem, diagnosis, type and frequency of therapy, future plans, and treatment goals. CHAMPUS has recently contracted with a utilization review service which must preapprove treatment of more than two sessions per week or more than 23 sessions per year. Even if services are approved by their utilization review intermediary, CHAMPUS still reserves the right to refuse payment. Inpatient care is generally limited to 60 days per calendar year unless a waiver is granted. New legislation was being considered during the preparation of this book that could lead to more benefit limits.

Fees are based on a UCR system. Some deductibles apply. Dependents of active duty personnel usually have a 20% co-payment, while other CHAMPUS patients have a 25% co-payment.

Participation by providers in the CHAMPUS program is voluntary, and the decision regarding participation can be made on a case-by-case basis. CHAMPUS has a reputation for being slow to pay. Although CHAMPUS UCR rates previously seemed reasonable, in the past 5 years they have lagged well behind inflation through freezes and other subtle mechanisms.

In several locales where there are large numbers of military personnel, CHAMPUS has contracted managed-care arrangements. Practitioners negotiate directly with the contractor to provide services for set fees. CHAMPUS has also established various demonstration programs that may have implications not only for the entire CHAMPUS system, but for federal programs as a whole.

As with other programs, the initial payment of a claim does not guarantee final acceptance. *Psychotherapy Finances* ("CHAMPUS: How Poor Records," 1990) reports the case of a licensed counselor who was forced into bankruptcy when CHAMPUS demanded that $587,000 in previously paid benefits be returned. Although CHAMPUS initially paid several years of claims, all were subsequently denied. According to the report, the counselor was part of a five-therapist clinic that was flagrantly flouting the CHAMPUS requirement for physician referral and kept very poor records. Government and insurance companies can demand restitution of claims that are paid and subsequently denied.

FEDERAL EMPLOYEES HEALTH BENEFITS PROGRAM (FEHB)

The Federal Employees Health Benefits Act created funding for federal employee group health plans. Although more than 10 million federal employees are enrolled in plans meeting these guidelines, there are hundreds of participating plans and options (Stromberg et al., 1988).

All these plans allow direct access to a clinical psychologist without supervision by a physician. Outpatient mental health services are usually reimbursed at 80%, while 100% of inpatient services are usually paid. HMOs and independent practice organizations are exempt and not required to include psychologists as participating providers or to reimburse for services provided by psychologists. These plans are administered by a variety of carriers.

In 1990, based on recommendations of a federal commission, U.S. Representative Gary Ackerman introduced legislative action to overhaul the FEHB program. His proposals included a two-option plan with the High Option covering 75% of the cost of up to 50 mental health visits and 90% of unlimited inpatient days. The Standard Option would cover 75% of the cost of up to 25 mental health visits and 80% of the cost of unlimited inpatient days. This plan would also continue the option of an HMO alternative. The bill was not passed. Representative Ackerman plans to introduce a revised bill revamping FEHB in 1991 ("Move to Change," 1990).

CHAPTER 8
OTHER THIRD-PARTY FUNDING SOURCES

There are numerous private and governmental sources that pay for the services of private practicing mental health professionals. These include corporations and governmental agencies that screen employees for sensitive positions (such as nuclear power plants, prisons, and child care); courts and attorneys who request child custody and other forensic evaluations; and various human service agencies who utilize mental health consultants. Several of these sources will be discussed in this chapter.

EMPLOYEE ASSISTANCE PLANS

Employee Assistance Plans (EAPs) were developed in the 1970s and have proliferated over the intervening years. In 1986, 50% to 60% of Fortune 500 companies had operating EAPs (Wise, 1988). It is likely that the number now approaches, or perhaps exceeds, 90%.

Interestingly, EAPs have grown by demonstrating to corporate executives that mental health treatment reduces absenteeism, hospital utilization, and tardiness and that it improves productivity. Although many employers have embraced EAPs, they have not typically increased (and have often cut back) the mental health component of their group insurance plans.

EAPs may be run by large national management companies, local hospital-based organizations, or individual practices. EAP personnel generally offer a variety of services to businesses, including management consultation, seminars, and assessment and referral services. The latter function provides ready access to a counselor (at no charge to the employee) for a limited number of sessions (usually between three and eight) and referral to another professional if further counseling is necessary.

EAPS provide mental health professionals opportunities for both direct work within the EAP and referrals from the EAP. Many EAPs hire mental health professionals to provide assessment and referral services. In order to avoid a possible conflict of interest, some require the EAP provider to refer any employee needing treatment beyond the initial allotment of sessions to another therapist. Others offer to pay practitioners a very low fee for the initial EAP sessions and allow the same practitioners to charge their full fee when employees continue treatment beyond the number of sessions stipulated by the EAP. The ethics of this situation may be questionable.

Through its EAP, a corporation typically pays for the initial allotment of sessions. Further sessions are the responsibility of the patient and insurance company. However, some employers will provide a partial or full subsidy, even for sessions beyond the initial ones, with the approval of the EAP representative.

Most EAPs emphasize substance abuse treatment. EAP professional literature, leaders in the field, and EAP promotional materials all stress substance abuse and its adverse impact on an employee's well-being and productivity. Those working as EAP counselors should be comfortable with this emphasis.

Some EAP counselors are employees of the corporations they serve. Others work for companies that contract with the target corporations. EAP counselors often like to refer to individuals with discrete specialties, such as child or sex therapy; or to those with a specific attraction, such as lower fees or Saturday hours. A therapist should be comfortable working with the EAP counselor who may want to continue involvement with the patient and may see himself or herself as a co-therapist, or even a continuing overseer and critic of the therapy. Issues of confidentiality must be carefully addressed.

WORKERS' COMPENSATION, VOCATIONAL REHABILITATION, AND SOCIAL SECURITY

There are numerous opportunities for mental health professionals to work with individuals who have been disabled through work, automobile accidents, or other situations. Services may include both assessment and treatment.

Psychologists and psychiatrists are eligible to perform evaluations for Social Security, which is usually administered through state agencies. The fees are generally set by the state and their attractiveness varies from state to state.

Therapists wishing to specialize as private sector rehabilitation counselors are referred to an article by Dvonch (1990).

Virtually all states require employers to insure their employees for work-related injuries. Workers' compensation insurance is often privately issued, although subject to governmental regulations. Mental health practitioners may be eligible to evaluate and/or treat people under workers' compensation. State laws vary regarding which professions are recognized to provide workers' compensation services. Insurance companies may allow payment to a psychologist or social worker even when the prevailing state law does not require such coverage.

A drawback with accepting workers' compensation cases is the fact that they are often subject to lengthy litigation. Many patients cannot afford to pay a mental health professional in advance for services that may later be paid in full by the workers' compensation insurance. Unfortunately, it sometimes takes years before these cases are settled and the practitioner may then discover that the services are ineligible for payment.

AUTOMOBILE INSURANCE

Most states require drivers to carry some minimum amount of personal accident insurance. The automobile insurer becomes the primary payer in automobile injury cases, and only when the automobile policy coverage runs out does the accident victim's health insurance take over. Mental health services are often paid in full but subject to the same potential difficulties as were noted in the discussion on workers' compensation. In Pennsylvania, therapists can receive only 110% of what Medicare would pay. Insurance companies perform their own reviews and decide what is appropriate treatment, whether it is accident related, and what is a reasonable fee. If victims are dissatisfied with the insurance company's payment, it becomes their burden (or perhaps the service provider's), to pursue payment, often through litigation.

CRIME VICTIM PROGRAMS

Many states have developed programs, often funded through fines and restitution fees, to assist the victims of criminal acts. These usually provide full or partial assistance for psychotherapy and medical costs that are not covered by insurance or other subsidies. The programs rarely guarantee payment in advance and delays can be long. Interested therapists should contact the Attorney General in their state to find out if such programs exist and request copies of applicable rules and guidelines.

HEALTH CARE FACILITIES

Most individuals providing mental health services in a hospital setting are either salaried employees of the hospital or they operate as independent practitioners and bill the patient or insurance company for the services provided. Another alternative is to contract with the hospital, so that the hospital bills the insurance company or patient for the independent practitioners' services and pays the practitioner on an independent contractor, fee-for-service basis.

Allowing hospitals to bill for your services can have major advantages in dealing with Blue Cross/Blue Shield. Although therapist services are usually billed to Blue Shield, the hospital may be able to gain more reimbursement through Blue Cross. Through an increased *per diem* or other means, the hospital may recoup the practitioner's fee plus additional administrative costs for itself. The advantage to the practitioner is that reimbursement may be higher and the hospital does virtually all of the administrative work. Since each Blue Cross/Blue Shield organization is different and insurance plans are changing so quickly, it would be necessary to carefully investigate this option and its possible applicability in your specific situation.

Nursing homes are an oft-neglected area with mental health services. These services include psychological evaluations, counseling of patients and families, and assistance to nursing home personnel in the management of difficult patients. Previously, all incoming nursing home residents were required to be screened by psychiatrists. Recent regulations have expanded the screeners to other "qualified mental health professionals." HCFA has not yet defined which practitioners will be included (Youngstrom, 1990).

CHAPTER 9
MANAGED CARE

Although virtually every issue of *Psychiatric News, The American Psychological Association Monitor*, and other professional newspapers has articles on *managed care*, the term is rarely defined. Wiggins (1989a) calls it a "global concept purported to control costs of health services provided in group plans sponsored by employers" (p. 12), including HMOs, PPOs, and fee-for-service plans with perspective review of hospital stays. Small (1989) says it "is not a legal term, but seems to refer to any plan which attempts to control the cost of health care by setting limits on reimbursement" (p. 12). Rascati (personal communication, March 27, 1990) gives one of the best definitions of managed care as "any program or service which attempts to direct or influence the use of medical care resources for an individual patient in advance of or during the course of care." Managed care is most often used to describe any plan, especially an HMO or PPO, that takes an active role in cost containment. Indemnity insurance plans that require prospective review of hospital stays or outpatient care are also generally included under definitions of managed care. In fact, insurance companies have always done some utilization review and made an effort to contain costs through payment limitations; but until the past few years, these attempts have not been widespread.

The managed-care concept has taken the health care industry by storm. In 1982, managed care accounted for only 2% of commercial insurers' business (Stromberg et al., 1988). In 1981, only 4% of all group enrollees were in capitated plans (Wiggins, 1989a). Two-year-old predictions that by 1992, 70% of Americans will receive health care through managed care (Berkman, Bassos, & Post, 1988), seemed fulfilled early when Herrington (1990) reported that 40% were already covered by managed indemnity plans, 20% in HMOs, and another 20% in PPOs. With health care costs accounting for an increasing percentage of the Gross National Product and becoming particularly onerous for employers, it is likely that trends towards drastic decreases in traditional fee-for-service plans, as well as more employee cost sharing, will continue.

HEALTH MAINTENANCE ORGANIZATIONS

Although *health maintenance organizations (HMOs)* were first established more than 50 years ago, their significance rose after the 1960s. In 1970, there were approximately 30 HMOs serving 3 million individuals. By 1986, there were over 400 HMOs serving 20 million people. It is estimated that in the early 1990s, more than 700 HMOs will serve 70 million subscribers (Frankel, 1990; Stromberg et al., 1988).

HMOs began in the 1930s as prepaid group practice plans. Among the largest and most successful was the Kaiser-Permanente Program in California. There were also other small plans. HMOs received significant support in the early 1970s when they were promoted as a "true health system," as opposed to the traditional "sickness system." The Health Maintenance Organization Act was enacted in 1973. This act preempted state restrictions on HMOs and provided federal grants and loans for those meeting federal guidelines (Frankel, 1990).

The 1973 law required employers of 25 or more persons, who offer a group health plan, to also offer employees an opportunity to enroll in a federally qualified HMO. Such plans had to provide a specific, comprehensive set of services, including inpatient hospitalization, crisis intervention, and at least 20 mental health outpatient visits. Federally qualified HMOs could not refuse enrollment or expel subscribers because of their health status, had to set premiums based on community ratings (rather than individual qualities), and follow other regulations.

Federal qualification was originally more important because of federal financial support and the eligibility for Medicare. As government financial support has disappeared and Medicare conditions for HMO participation have been broadened, many HMOs have successfully developed without federal qualification.

HMOs can be organized along several models. In *staff HMOs* (such as Kaiser-Permanente) the HMO employs providers full-time to see only HMO enrollees. Interestingly, Kaiser-Permanente broke precedent in 1990 by using part-time independently contracted psychological providers, apparently because of an employee shortage.

Under a *group HMO* plan, providers are incorporated into a group that contracts with the HMO on a *capitation basis* (i.e., providers are paid a fixed fee per enrollee, regardless of how much service is provided).

The largest and fastest growing types of HMOs involve *independent practice associations (IPAs)* or hybrid IPA/group plans. One common form involves primary providers (e.g., family practitioners, gynecologists, pediatricians) who are paid on a capitated basis, while referral services (e.g., surgeons, psychologists, psychiatrists) are paid on a fee-for-service basis. The HMO contracts with the individual mental health provider. Services are reimbursed based on a previously agreed schedule of charges, which is usually lower than prevailing fees. Frequently, a portion of the reimbursement (often around 15%) is withheld and placed in a "shared risk pool." At the end of the year, all providers receive a portion (0% to 100%) of payments previously withheld, depending on the HMO's final balance sheet. Some HMOs reserve the right to charge providers even more than the withheld percentage in an especially unprofitable year. Providers in IPA models usually practice in their own offices and see both HMO and non-HMO patients.

Several HMOs have used the capitation model for mental health services. Biodyne is a mental health corporation that has large contracts in California, Hawaii, and other states, solely to provide mental health services. These HMOs are paid a set fee per enrollee which covers all outpatient and inpatient costs.

Other large HMOs provide no direct mental health services and instead contract the entire mental health segment of their care. The mental health contractor may then subcontract to other groups, who in turn may subcontract several more times. The impact of several levels of subcontractors significantly reduces the hourly reimbursement received by the ultimate service provider. The actual therapist is often reimbursed only $15 to $30 per hour. These fees tend to attract therapists with lesser credentials or those starting a practice. Not unlike the phenomena seen in public mental health centers, lower reimbursement rates may lead to pressure for high volume and may result in a high turnover of therapists.

The concept of HMOs sounds appealing. By paying practitioners to maintain health rather than to treat sickness, HMOs try to encourage prevention and early intervention. In reality, just as indemnity systems can be criticized for encouraging overutilization of services, HMOs often discourage appropriate utilization of services, to the patient's detriment.

HMOs have been criticized for subjecting patients to long waits for appointments, reducing availability of hospital care and specialists, and excluding nonphysician mental health providers from the referral pool. Studies suggest that HMOs do not contain health cost, put conflict-of-interest pressures on physicians, take mostly the healthiest employees, and charge the same rates as carriers who serve higher risk populations (Buie, 1987, 1988, 1989a).

HMOs are often accused of treating therapists as "commodities" and of appreciating practitioners only for the "market value" of their degrees, with little regard for their clinical skills, professionalism, or dedication.

A major criticism of the mental health care provided by HMOs is that it overemphasizes short-term psychotherapy, to the exclusion of long-term treatment. This emphasis not only affects therapists with psychodynamic practices, but also most other practitioners. For example, many plans limit outpatient sessions to 20 per year, regardless of individual circumstances. If a therapist is seeing a depressed patient with suicidal potential, but who is clearly manageable on an outpatient basis, this individual might need to be seen at least once or twice a week during a crisis period. Managing the crisis could easily consume half the yearly allotment in a month or 6 weeks.

PREFERRED PROVIDER ORGANIZATIONS AND PROFESSIONAL PROVIDER ARRANGEMENTS

Preferred Provider Organizations (PPOs) are actually a variant of HMOs, similar to the IPA model. In fact, because the PPO is more of an arrangement than an organization, it is frequently being referred to as a *Professional Provider Arrangement (PPA)*.

In a PPO, the subscriber is given a financial incentive to utilize a select panel of preferred providers. For example, subscribers might be entitled to 80% or 100% reimbursement for psychotherapy with PPO panelists, but only 50% with nonpanelists. The

PPO contracts with providers and generally negotiates a reduced fee. In return, participating providers supposedly receive increased volume and rapid claims processing. Providers also agree to utilization review, often quite rigorous, which provides cost control. PPOs usually do not have a "shared risk pool."

The difference between HMOs and PPOs is not always distinct. PPOs have been sponsored by provider groups (e.g., hospitals, physicians, other health professionals) as well as insurance companies, self-insured employers, or private third-party administrators.

Classes of providers can be included or eliminated through the PPO structure. For example, eligibility for a hospital-based PPO might require membership on the active medical staff. If psychologists and social workers are not eligible for full hospital privileges, they will not be allowed on the PPO panel. These arrangements are not usually affected by state Freedom of Choice laws because PPOs are not insurance companies. On the other hand, several states have enacted, or are in the process of establishing, legislation that might affect PPO membership.

Criticisms of PPOs often depend on the specific type. Employers sometimes view provider-based PPOs skeptically because of fears that they will not rigorously control costs. Physician-based and hospital-based PPOs have been accused of excluding classes of providers such as psychologists and social workers.

PPOs established by insurance companies or third-party administrators are subject to many of the same criticisms as HMOs. They are often accused of valuing profits over good patient care. Both practitioners and patients often believe that PPO regulations are overly restrictive.

JOINING AN HMO OR PPO

Mental health practitioners are increasingly invited to join HMOs, PPOs, and other referral panels and networks. When invited, it is important to read the contract carefully and to consider all the implications of one's decision on whether to become a member. Among the considerations are:

1. *Initiation Fee* - The organization may require an amount ranging from $25 to several thousand dollars. Even small fees become significant losses if a practitioner joins 8 or 10 organizations and receives no patients. There seem to be a number of organizations of questionable credibility, which offer to place a therapist on a preferred provider panel, but rarely or never provide referrals.
2. *Term of the Contract* - Some contracts allow withdrawal by either party with 30 days' notice, others on a yearly anniversary date. As therapists usually agree to see all patients from that organization, they should carefully consider the contract terms. Some beginning practitioners have joined HMOs and PPOs that have exceptionally low reimbursement rates. As their practices have grown, the therapists find themselves busy and resent seeing patients at 50% or less of their standard fee. As the HMO/PPO practice has filled all available hours, these therapists have not had time to see other private patients.
3. *Provider Compensation* - HMOs and PPOs may negotiate a different fee with each provider, have a standard reimbursement schedule, or ask for a particular

discount from a therapist's regular fee. Practitioners are often asked to accept a "prevailing fee," which they may later be surprised to find is much lower than what they expected. It is important to note the patient's co-payment and whether the PPO or HMO is required to pay the therapist within a specified number of days (and what penalty is incurred if it does not). Practitioners also should note any percentage being withheld for a shared risk pool and *not* make financial calculations based on the assumption that they will eventually receive most or all these withheld monies.

4. *Covered Services* - It is crucial to examine how many psychotherapy sessions are allowed for each patient and what services are covered (such as psychological testing, biofeedback, or hypnotherapy). If a noncovered service is provided, can the practitioner bill the patient? A therapist should probably not sign a contract that does not include the practitioner's usual services, or limits him or her to providing far less than is usual. For example, a psychoanalytically oriented practitioner who sees all patients at least once a week is likely to be very unhappy with a plan allowing only 20 sessions per year. Although many plans allow the practitioner to collect from the patient for services over and above the limits, patients generally feel entitled to full coverage and resent paying anything beyond the prescribed co-payment.

5. *Utilization Review* - The practitioner should carefully examine the procedures used by the HMO/PPO to review one's services. How often are telephone calls and written reports required? What recourse does a practitioner have if the reviewer turns down the service? How much time and effort is likely to be involved in utilization review?

6. *Referral Arrangements* - HMOs and PPOs often encourage or require providers to refer patients only to other providers participating in that particular HMO or PPO. If mental health practitioners are not comfortable with the other participants, they may not wish to join. On the other hand, if they respect most of the panel members, enrollment may provide more opportunity to receive referrals from compatible practitioners in other fields.

In summary, the possible advantages of joining an HMO or PPO include access to more patients and simplified payment. Disadvantages include a lower hourly fee, pressure for shorter terms of therapy, various constraints on practice, and increased paperwork and administrative difficulties. Detailed lists of questions one might ask before joining a PPO are found in Frankel (1990) and Stromberg et al. (1988).

PRACTICAL ISSUES

Managed-care organizations can be rather arbitrary. Some limit coverage only to acute crisis interventions. Others may exclude "personality disorders" or even chronic anxiety states. Telephone reviewers may have limited qualifications and training and may make decisions based solely on simple arbitrary formulas. I had a patient with a history of long-term severe drug abuse, serious victimization, and a host of other psychological trauma and self-destructive behaviors. The presenting problem was anxiety, which improved. Despite several major life events that were currently occurring and were increasing both her anxiety and vulnerability to severe decompensation, the telephone reviewer rudely refused further treatment. A great deal of time and effort put into follow-up phone calls and letters had no impact (Small, 1989). Unfortunately, such tales are growing increasingly common.

Interestingly, managed-care reviewers are often "fourth parties" (separate utilization review companies hired by PPOs, HMOs, and insurance companies). Therapists have reported spending up to an hour on the telephone to gain approval for as few as three sessions. These cost management firms "prove their worth" to employers by how much they reduce utilization. Thus, their incentive may be cost containment rather than patient care. Often, adversarial relationships seem to emerge in which the reviewers are accused of treating professionals in the same way IRS auditors are often accused of treating taxpayers (i.e., assuming the practitioner is "trying to get away with something").

In a utilization review, a nonmental-health specialist will typically consider the provider's request for an initial three or four sessions. These are often approved fairly routinely. By the end of these sessions, the therapist will complete a multipage treatment plan and/or have one or more telephone reviews with a psychiatric nurse, psychologist, or psychiatrist. If the plan is approved, six or seven more sessions may be authorized. Ethical problems when a therapist disagrees with a utilization review were discussed in Chapter 4.

The health care reimbursement picture has undergone permanent changes. No longer will unrestricted reimbursement along a UCR model predominate. One can expect various hybrids of HMOs and PPOs, probably involving more choices for consumers, more pressure on practitioners, and more administrative burdens. Many might agree with Kovacs (1987b) that psychologists (and perhaps social workers and other therapists) should leave the health service arena and become separate human service professionals, supporting themselves only with consumer fees. Otherwise, it is essential that one actively keep informed of rapidly changing developments in the area of managed care.

CHAPTER 10
CURRENT AND FUTURE TRENDS

NATIONAL HEALTH INSURANCE

Since the 1970s, national health insurance has been predicted to be "around the corner" ("National Health Plans," 1979). Senator Edward Kennedy's name has been closely identified with bills to establish national health insurance for 20 years. The 1988 presidential campaign highlighted the large number of citizens who are not eligible for Medicaid or Medicare and who also have no health insurance. It seems almost inevitable that the problems of the uninsured will eventually be subject to legislation, probably at a federal level. This legislation may involve a federally subsidized pool to provide insurance to all United States citizens or a true plan of national health insurance.

If national health insurance becomes a reality, it may continue to operate within the framework of the existing private insurance system. It currently seems unlikely that the United States will adopt plans similar to the Canadian or British health care systems. In any case, federal guidelines will probably mandate that all insurance plans have specified coverage. A method would be developed to insure that all citizens receive coverage (e.g., an assigned risk pool). Another possibility would be a federally administered health insurance system, perhaps similar to Medicare. The more radical the program, the more time it is likely to take to enact.

DRUG AND ALCOHOL TREATMENT

During the 1980s, the importance of treatment for substance abuse was recognized and amply reimbursed. Many states passed laws requiring insurance plans to cover alcohol and/or drug abuse treatment. The 28-day inpatient stay became the standard of care.

In the last few years, insurance companies have increasingly balked at allowing long inpatient stays ("Will Companies Cut," 1989). Research has questioned whether inpatient treatment has any advantage over outpatient treatment (D. O'Connell, personal communication, February 13, 1991). Insurance companies reimbursement policies are encouraging short inpatient detoxification, more outpatient treatment, and less inpatient care.

It is likely that preferential treatment for substance abuse, as opposed to mental health problems, will continue. On the other hand, insurance companies will continue their critical evaluation of options for substance abuse treatment and will probably continue to prefer outpatient services.

DIAGNOSIS RELATED GROUPS (DRGS), PROSPECTIVE PAYMENT, RELATIVE VALUE SCALES (RVS), AND INDEMNITY

In order to cut costs, Medicare passed a law in 1983 which provided fixed payments to hospitals for inpatient stays based on particular Diagnosis Related Groups (DRGs). The idea was to reverse the traditional situation in which hospitals had financial incentives for keeping people in the hospital longer and filling empty beds. DRGs were discussed in detail in Chapter 7.

Other programs and private insurers quickly adopted this *prospective payment system*. Although DRGs have not yet been widely applied to outpatient treatment, managed-care programs are increasingly scrutinizing outpatient treatment before authorizing payment and often are requiring prior approval. It would not be surprising if, in a few years, insurance companies began authorizing differential numbers of outpatient sessions depending on a patient's diagnosis.

A more likely possibility is that *Relative Value Scales (RVSs)* will be utilized (Wiggins, 1988c, 1989b). Various medical organizations, the federal government, and insurance companies are studying "appropriate" weightings for different medical procedures. To date, most RVS studies have indicated that surgery procedures are "overvalued" (i.e., currently paid at too high a rate compared to other services) and "cognitive" procedures such as diagnostic office visits with an internist are "undervalued." If RVS systems are enacted, it seems possible that psychological and psychiatric procedures may receive somewhat higher relative values in the future than they currently receive.

BIOLOGICAL VERSUS MENTAL ILLNESSES

For many years, insurance companies have reimbursed nonpsychiatric medical services at a much higher rate than psychiatric services. Some neuropsychological examiners have found that when an *ICD-9 psychiatric* diagnosis for organic brain syndrome is used, payment is considerably less than when they specify a similar *ICD-9 neurological* diagnosis.

Several suits have been initiated against insurance companies, charging them with providing discriminatory reimbursement for beneficiaries treated for bipolar illnesses and claiming that the reimbursement should be equivalent to other physical illnesses ("Bipolar Disorder," 1988; "California Mandates Parity," 1989; "Court Rulings," 1989; "Suit Filed," 1990). A California law went into effect in 1990 which mandates individuals with "schizophrenia, schizo-affective disorder, bipolar disorder, delusional depression and pervasive development disorder" to have the same coverage as would be provided for other physical illnesses. The proliferation of lawsuits and legislation challenging differential reimbursement based on diagnosis may significantly affect the traditional distinction between mental and physical disorders. It may also further exacerbate tension between the psychiatric community and nonphysician providers.

PEER REVIEW

Although *Peer review* was the hot concept of the early 1980s, it has since dropped out of sight. Both the American Psychiatric Association and the American Psychological Association set up programs to monitor appropriate utilization of mental health services for insurance companies. Because professional organizations provided these services, they tended to be patient-oriented and perhaps too lenient with providers. The gentle guidance and mild limit-setting of peer review has been replaced with the harsher controls of managed-care utilization review.

FUTURE TRENDS

The days of "provider-driven" reimbursement schedules are probably over. The average cost per employee enrolled in a group health plan jumped from $1,724 in 1985 to $2,745 in 1989 (Goldman, 1990). As health care costs continue to outstrip inflation, most third-party reimbursement plans will aggressively pursue cost containment.

America may be moving toward a "three-tiered" or even "four-tiered" health care system. The poorest segment of the population will continue to be covered by medical assistance plans. These plans will probably remain underfunded, despite the increased demands caused by AIDS and other health problems, as well as economic and social forces. Adequate mental health coverage on a national scale is unlikely.

The severely mentally ill will continue to obtain medicine, and those who are dangerous or seriously nonfunctional will obtain care through public facilities. Clinicians interested in serving these populations will usually be employed by state hospitals and mental health centers. Salaries will be moderate. There will be little opportunity for independent practitioners to serve the indigent.

There is increasing concern about the "near-poor," those citizens who are unable to afford health insurance, have low-paying jobs, and are still ineligible for public assistance. This problem will probably be addressed either through expansion of Medicaid (with small premiums for this group), "bare bones" mandatory coverage, or vouchers which may operate like food stamps. In any case, it is unlikely that these individuals will be able to receive many mental health services outside of the already overburdened public clinics.

Among those with private insurance, there are likely to be two levels of health care. Employers will cope with increasing health care costs by making employees pay a larger share of their health insurance premiums. Larger companies will offer a choice of coverage. Most workers will probably opt for lower premiums and will accept restrictions as to which providers they can see as well as the additional constraints of managed care. The "top tier" will insist on freedom to see providers of their choice and will pay for this privilege.

Even those accepting managed care will increasingly demand more options. Patients will be given moderate incentives to use participating providers but will still receive some reimbursement when they select nonparticipating providers. Heavy pressure will be exerted on providers to cut their fees.

It is unclear whether mental health benefits will decline, increase, or remain the same. Employees choosing "lower tier" plans will have limited benefits. After many of these workers and their families face mental health problems, more demand may arise for adequate mental health coverage.

Traditional rivalries among professions will continue. Psychiatrists will emphasize "biological" illnesses and demand reimbursement equivalent to other medical illnesses. As psychologists begin to obtain full hospital privileges as well as limited rights to prescribe medication, and as the number of nondoctoral level therapists increases, psychologists and psychiatrists will probably increasingly find themselves as allies. Nurses, mental health counselors, and other therapists will compete with psychologists and psychiatrists by offering lower fees and will increasingly obtain insurance and managed-care reimbursement. Masters-level social workers will find themselves in the middle. Some managed-care organizations will try to limit costs by reimbursing only psychiatrists and perhaps psychologists. Others will continue to develop subcontracts in which physicians and psychologists may be supervisors of providers with more limited credentials who are providing the actual clinical services at a lower fee.

Cost containment will also be effected through government regulations. Medicare and other federal programs will bravely attempt to keep health care cost increases at, or below, inflation. They will probably continue to fail in their cost-containment efforts, as hospitals provide more expensive technology and physicians perform more procedures. Although cost per procedure may not increase (and may even decrease), the number and types of procedures will probably continue to go up. Unfortunately, mental health practitioners who only charge for their time may find themselves increasingly squeezed by the cost-containment movement. Those doing only therapy will find themselves working more hours for less money. Psychiatrists may be able to keep up with inflation by dispensing their own medications (like many internists and family and general practitioners), scheduling short medication review sessions, and providing more hospital-based services and consultations.

Psychologists may find fewer alternatives for maximizing payments for their time. Testing procedures may proliferate, but insurance companies have not usually been generous in reimbursing for these services. Like psychiatrists, they may find themselves hired by agencies that require a doctoral-level professional for work with certain clients, but which have most actual clinical work performed by less credentialed (e.g., masters- and bachelor-level) staff.

The most ominous trend is the growing tendency to mandate fees. In several states, fees for specific services have been tied to Medicare. For example, a 1990 Pennsylvania law states that medical (and mental health) providers cannot charge auto accident victims more than 110% of what Medicare will pay for a service or, if there is no Medicare rate, more than 80% of the practitioner's usual fee. This law not only disallows insurance payments of more than those amounts, but also requires the provider to charge the patient no more than those amounts, even if the patient is willing to pay the full fee.

Other laws mandate that providers cannot charge an individual who is eligible for Medicare any more than what Medicare accepts as a reasonable fee. If these legislative trends continue, it is possible that the government will eventually mandate maximum fees for all health services.

Another interesting trend involves "rationing" of health care resources. In its Medicaid program, Oregon became the first state to set priorities for health care payments, balancing the cost of treatment against expected benefits (Egan, 1990). At the current time, this approach eliminates only a few expensive high-technology procedures; however, one should expect considerations of cost-benefit ratios to be applied to more government and private programs. The actual impact on mental health services is unclear, yet pessimism is justified. Despite many studies showing the cost benefits of preventive mental health services (American Psychological Association, undated-b; Frisman, McGuire, & Rosenbach, 1985; McGuire, 1981), psychotherapy is often the first service to be cut in cost-containment efforts.

As is obvious from my previous comments, I believe mental health care reimbursement is undergoing major changes. Although doomsayers predict the demise of independent practice, I would suggest that the "golden age" of private mental health practice probably never existed. Before the 1970s, only psychiatrists were reimbursed for most mental health services, and many policies offered no mental health coverage. The 1970s and 1980s saw increasing numbers of eligible providers and more private practitioners emerging in a variety of disciplines. Despite an expansion in the number of policies offering mental health coverage, the proportion of fees covered by those policies often decreased.

The 1990s will bring increasing cost containment, utilization review, and managed care. Pressure will be exerted to provide more services for less money, a serious threat to optimal care. However, these efforts will be counterbalanced by patients who will seek out caregivers with the expertise and willingness to spend the time necessary to help resolve their problems. Despite the "corporatization" of health care, it is likely that ethical and competent independent practitioners who are willing to stay informed and adapt to change will continue to thrive.

APPENDICES

APPENDIX A
OFFICE MANAGEMENT PRODUCTS AND SOFTWARE

OFFICE MANAGEMENT PRODUCTS

The following companies are some of the better known suppliers of Health Care Financing Administration (HCFA) insurance forms, personalized statements, super-bills, and numerous other office management products. Specifically request their *medical* catalogs.

Colwell Systems, Inc., 201 Kenyon Road, P.O. Box 4024, Champaign, IL 61824-4024. Telephone: 1-800-225-1448.

HISTACOUNT, 965 Walt Whitman Road, Melville, NY 11747. Telephone: 1-516-421-1200.

Medical Arts Press, 3440 Winnetaha Avenue, North, Minneapolis, MN 55427. Telephone: 1-800-826-6706.

Moore Business Products, P.O. Box 5000, Vernon Hills, IL 60061. Telephone: 1-800-323-6230.

The Overheadshrinkers, P.O. Box 3677, South Pasadena, CA 91031. Telephone: 1-818-799-6882.

Sycom, Inc., West Beltline Highway, P.O. Box 7947, Madison, WI 53707-7947. Telephone: 1-800-356-8141.

UAL Medical Products, P.O. Box 1265, Whittier, CA 90610. Telephone: 1-800-992-5755.

OFFICE MANAGEMENT SOFTWARE

The following companies offer some of the more widely used software (i.e., computer programs) for managing a mental health practice. All of the listed programs do bookkeeping and produce patient statements, insurance forms, and numerous practice management reports. All can provide you with descriptive literature, nominally priced demonstration disks, and a reference list of some of their current users.

IN-SITE Billing System and Multi-Provider Billing System (MPB). AI Software, Inc., P.O. Box 724, Wakefield, RI 02880-0724. Telephone: 1-800-272-2250.

Mental Health Office Manager (MHOM). Synergistic Office Solutions, Inc., 4801 S. University Drive, Suite 305, Davie, FL 33328. Telephone: 1-305-434-2207.

SHRINK: The Practice Manager. Multi-Health Systems, 908 Niagara Falls Boulevard, North Tonawanda, NY 14120-2060. Telephone: 1-800-456-3003. Multi-Health Systems, 65 Overlea Boulevard, Suite 210, Toronto, Ontario, Canada M4H 1P1. Psychological Assessment Resources, Inc., P.O. Box 998, Odessa, FL 33556. Telephone: 1-800-331-8378.

WPS Logical Patient Billing System. Western Psychological Services, 12031 Wilshire Boulevard, Los Angeles, CA 90025. Telephone: 1-800-648-8857.

APPENDIX B
COMPUTER GENERATED INSURANCE FORMS, PATIENT STATEMENTS, AND PRACTICE MANAGEMENT REPORTS

This section includes samples of a limited selection of the forms and reports produced by Mental Health Office Manager (MHOM). Practice management software from other vendors (listed in Appendix A) produces similar reports.

These forms/reports have been reduced slightly for inclusion in this book. They can be printed on either continuous word processing and computer paper or single sheets of letter-size paper.

All names used are fictitious and any similarities to actual persons, living or dead, are purely coincidental.

Administrative Services
123 Broadway
New York City, NY 11122

FORM APPROVED
OMB NO. 0938-0008

HEALTH INSURANCE CLAIM FORM
(CHECK APPLICABLE PROGRAM BLOCK BELOW)

☐ MEDICARE (MEDICARE NO.)	☐ MEDICAID (MEDICAID NO.)	☐ CHAMPUS (SPONSOR'S SSN)	☐ CHAMPVA (VA FILE NO.)	☐ FECA BLACK LUNG (SSN)	☐ OTHER (CERTIFICATE SSN)

PATIENT AND INSURED (SUBSCRIBER) INFORMATION

1. PATIENT'S NAME (LAST NAME, FIRST NAME, MIDDLE INITIAL)	2. PATIENT'S DATE OF BIRTH	3. INSURED'S NAME (LAST NAME, FIRST NAME, MIDDLE INITIAL)
Baldson Olaf	01 | 14 | 1963	Baldson, J.P.V.D.

4. PATIENT'S ADDRESS (STREET, CITY, STATE, ZIP CODE)	5. PATIENT'S SEX	6. INSURED'S I.D. NO. (FOR PROGRAM CHECKED ABOVE, INCLUDE ALL LETTERS)
6520 Ascerbic Cir. Hollywood, FL 33024	MALE [XX] FEMALE [ ]	B123-45-6789

TELEPHONE NO. (305)999-2222	7. PATIENT'S RELATIONSHIP TO INSURED	8. INSURED'S GROUP NO. (OR GROUP NAME OR FECA CLAIM NO.)
	SELF [ ] SPOUSE [ ] CHILD [XX] OTHER [ ]	U.P.D.A. ☐ INSURED IS EMPLOYED AND COVERED BY EMPLOYER HEALTH PLAN

9. OTHER HEALTH INSURANCE COVERAGE (ENTER NAME OF POLICYHOLDER AND PLAN NAME AND ADDRESS AND POLICY OR MEDICAL ASSISTANCE NUMBER)	10. WAS CONDITION RELATED TO:	11. INSURED'S ADDRESS (STREET, CITY, STATE, ZIP CODE)
Baldson, Ida Aetna P.O. Box 31450 Tampa, FL 33631-3450	A. PATIENT'S EMPLOYMENT YES [XX] NO [ ] B. ACCIDENT AUTO [ ] OTHER [ ]	6520 Ascerbic Cir. Hollywood, FL 33024 TELEPHONE NO. (305)999-2222

11.a. CHAMPUS SPONSOR'S
STATUS ☐ ACTIVE DUTY ☐ RETIRED ☐ DECEASED BRANCH OF SERVICE NONE

12. PATIENT'S OR AUTHORIZED PERSON'S SIGNATURE (READ BACK BEFORE SIGNING) I AUTHORIZE THE RELEASE OF ANY MEDICAL INFORMATION NECESSARY TO PROCESS THIS CLAIM. I ALSO REQUEST PAYMENT OF GOVERNMENT BENEFITS EITHER TO MYSELF OR TO THE PARTY WHO ACCEPTS ASSIGNMENT BELOW.	13. I AUTHORIZE PAYMENT OF MEDICAL BENEFITS TO UNDERSIGNED PHYSICIAN OR SUPPLIER FOR SERVICE DESCRIBED BELOW.
SIGNED SIGNATURE ON FILE DATE 09/01/89	SIGNATURE ON FILE SIGNED (INSURED OR AUTHORIZED PERSON)

PHYSICIAN OR SUPPLIER INFORMATION

14. DATE OF: ILLNESS (FIRST SYMPTOM) OR INJURY (ACCIDENT) OR PREGNANCY (LMP)	15. DATE FIRST CONSULTED YOU FOR THIS CONDITION 12/15/84	16. IF PATIENT HAS HAD SAME OR SIMILAR ILLNESS OR INJURY, GIVE DATES	16.a. IF EMERGENCY CHECK HERE ☐

17. DATE PATIENT ABLE TO RETURN TO WORK	18. DATES OF TOTAL DISABILITY FROM | THROUGH	DATES OF PARTIAL DISABILITY FROM | THROUGH

19. NAME OF REFERRING PHYSICIAN OR OTHER SOURCE (e.g. PUBLIC HEALTH AGENCY)	20. FOR SERVICES RELATED TO HOSPITALIZATION GIVE HOSPITALIZATION DATES
Marcus Welby, M.D. #12345	ADMITTED | DISCHARGED

21. NAME AND ADDRESS OF FACILITY WHERE SERVICES RENDERED (IF OTHER THAN HOME OR OFFICE)	22. WAS LABORATORY WORK PERFORMED OUTSIDE YOUR OFFICE?
NONE	YES [ ] NO [ ] CHARGES:

23. A. DIAGNOSIS OR NATURE OF ILLNESS OR INJURY. RELATE DIAGNOSIS TO PROCEDURE IN COLUMN D BY REFERENCE NUMBERS 1, 2, 3, ETC. OR DX CODE
1. 309.4
2.
3.
4. ICD-9 CM
24.

B. EPSDT YES [ ] NO [ ]
FAMILY PLANNING YES [ ] NO [ ]
PRIOR AUTHORIZATION NO.

A. DATE OF SERVICE FROM — TO	B. PLACE OF SERVICE	C. PROCEDURE CODE (IDENTIFY)	FULLY DESCRIBE PROCEDURES, MEDICAL SERVICES OR SUPPLIES FURNISHED FOR EACH DATE GIVEN (EXPLAIN UNUSUAL SERVICES OR CIRCUMSTANCES)	D. DIAGNOSIS CODE	E. CHARGES	F. DAYS OR UNITS	G. T.O.S.	H. LEAVE BLANK
08/23/89	3	90844	PSYCHOTHERAPY (1 HR)	309.4	100 | 00	1		12345
08/30/89	3	90844	PSYCHOTHERAPY (1 HR)	309.4	100 | 00	1		12345

25. SIGNATURE OF PHYSICIAN OR SUPPLIER (INCLUDING DEGREES(S) OR CREDENTIALS) (I CERTIFY THAT THE STATEMENTS ON THE REVERSE APPLY TO THIS BILL AND ARE MADE A PART THEREOF)	26. ACCEPT ASSIGNMENT (GOVERNMENT CLAIMS ONLY) (SEE BACK)	27. TOTAL CHARGE	28. AMOUNT PAID	29. BALANCE DUE
Katherine E. Peres, Ph.D.	YES [XX] NO [ ]	200 | 00		

DATE: 09/01/89	30. YOUR SOCIAL SECURITY NO.	31. PHYSICIAN'S, SUPPLIER'S, AND/OR GROUP NAME, ADDRESS, ZIP CODE AND TELEPHONE NO.
32. YOUR PATIENT'S ACCOUNT NO. 84180 (A)	33. YOUR EMPLOYER I.D. NO. 59-9999999	Pines Psychological Assoc. PA 4801 S. University Dr. #305 Davie, FL 33328 (305)434-2200 I.D. NO. J234567890

* PLACE OF SERVICE AND TYPE OF SERVICE (T.O.S.) CODES ON THE BACK
REMARKS:

APPROVED BY AMA COUNCIL ON MEDICAL SERVICE 5-83

Form **HCFA-1500** (C-1) (1-84)   Form **OWCP-1500**
Form **CHAMPUS-501**   Form **RRB-1500**

HCFA-1500 INSURANCE CLAIM FORM: The most common computer-generated claim format. Numerous other special and customized formats are available (e.g., to meet special state requirements, for primarily hospital practices, etc.).

```
                    Pines Psychological Associates, P.A.
                       4801 S. University Dr., Ste. 305
                             Davie, FL  33328

                          Telephone: (305)434-2200


     PATIENT NAME..: Lance Berkley
     ACCOUNT ID #..:  88078
     PATIENT D.O.B.: 12/10/71

     DATE OF SERVICE......: 10/22/90    PLACE/TYPE OF SERVICE CODES: 3  /
     LOCATION OF SERVICE..: Office
     SERVICE..............: INTAKE            CPT CODE: 90801
     FEE..................:      110.00
     ----------------------------------------------------------------------
                            INSURANCE INFORMATION

     ASSIGNMENT OF BENEFITS: I certify that the services listed have been
     received and I authorize payment be made to the provider named below.

                      Signed _____

     AUTHORIZATION TO RELEASE INFORMATION: I authorize the release of any
     privileged information necessary to process this claim.

                      Signed _____

     DIAGNOSIS: ICD-9
               1. 297.10    2.           3.           4.

     INSURED: Berkley, Lance          Policy #:74987173
     COMPANY: AV-MED Health Plan
     PT'S RELATIONSHIP TO INSURED: Self
     CONDITION RELATED TO EMPLOYMENT?: No    RELATED TO AN ACCIDENT?: No


                                          _____
               Provider's Signature.....:Seth R. Krieger, Ph.D.
                                          PY 0002882

               Supplier ID.............:84635-57874698
               Soc Sec or Empl ID #.....:59-2090881

     - - - - - - - - - - - - - - - - - - - - - - - - - - - - - - - - - - -
                       (Retain this portion for your Records)

                       Pines Psychological Associates, P.A.
                              PATIENT RECEIPT

     Name....:Lance Berkley                    Account #:88078
     Provider:Seth R. Krieger, Ph.D.           Date.....:10/22/90
     Service :INTAKE                           CPT Code.:90801
     Location:Office


                -Previous-   ----Fee----  --Payment--  -Adjustmnt-   New Balance
     Account...:    0.00       110.00        0.00         0.00         110.00
     Pt Portion:    0.00       110.00        0.00         0.00         110.00
     _____
     INSURANCE PATIENTS PLEASE NOTE: If expected insurance payments are denied,
     those charges will be added to your co-payment balance in future billing.
```

SUPERBILL: This computer-generated superbill serves as both a receipt and an insurance claim form to be submitted by the patient. Can be printed after each session.

```
Pines Psychological Associates, P.A.
4801 S. University Dr., Ste. 305
Davie, FL  33328


Jane Bowler                            Statement Date: 10/30/90
8021 NW 28th Place
Sunrise, FL 33322                      Page:  1


==================================================================
FOR PROFESSIONAL SERVICES RENDERED BY Katherine E. Peres, Ph.D.

Patient Name..: Jane Bowler
Account Number: 89023
Diagnosis.....: 302.73
                                    Previous Balance:      0.00
     --------------------------------------------------------------
     Date  Description                    Fee    Payment  Adjustment
     ----  -----------                  ------   -------  ----------
10/01/90 INTAKE            Check #2897  150.00   150.00
10/15/90 PSYCHOTHERAPY (1 HR)           100.00
10/22/90 PSYCHOTHERAPY (1 HR) Check #2907 100.00 100.00
10/29/90 PSYCHOTHERAPY (1 HR)           100.00
     --------------------------------------------------------------
       Account TOTALS...................  450.00   250.00     0.00

     --------------------------------------------------------------
    | Account Balance Now Due......................  $200.00  |
     --------------------------------------------------------------

==================================================================
***************** Thank you for your prompt payment! *********************


  --------------------------------------------------------------------
     Current       Over 30 Days    Over 60 Days    Over 90 Days
     -------       ------------    ------------    ------------
        0.00              0.00            0.00            0.00
```

```
INSURANCE PATIENTS PLEASE NOTE: If expected insurance payments are denied,
those charges will be added to your co-payment balance in future billing.
==================================================================
```

PATIENT STATEMENT: This computer-generated statement is one of several possible statement formats.

```
                                     Psychological Associates
   11/02/90                          OUTSTANDING INSURANCE REPORT                              Page   1
===================================================================================================================
        Insurance Name: AETNA                                  Note:Coverage MUST be confirmed
        Address.......: Reading, PA   19603                         before scheduling!
        Phone Number..: (800)544-2985
        Contact.......: Jade


                          TRANSACTION  FIRST    SECOND  DAYS            INS. PAYM       PROV
   ID        NAME             DATE     BILLED    BILLED UNITS   FEE     EXPECTED  CPT   CODE   COMMENT
 =======  ==============================  ========  ========  ======== ===== ========= ========= =======  == ===============
   90056 GREENJEANS, Laura   Pol#:249-56-0782         Grp#:                    Insured:Greenjeans, Ralph
                              9/18/90  10/04/90  10/04/90    1    120.00     120.00 90844       KP
                             10/02/90  10/04/90  10/04/90    1    120.00     120.00 90844       KP
                             10/09/90  10/15/90  10/15/90    1    120.00     120.00 90844       KP
                             10/16/90  11/02/90  11/02/90    1    120.00     120.00 90844       KP
                             10/23/90  11/02/90  11/02/90    1    120.00     120.00 90844       KP
                             10/30/90  11/02/90  11/02/90    1    120.00     120.00 90844       KP
                             ----------------------------------------------------------------
                           6 SERVICE(S)       PATIENT TOTAL:   720.00     720.00


 ===================================================================================================================
                           6 SERVICE(S)       INSURANCE TOTAL:  720.00     720.00
 ===================================================================================================================
        Insurance Name: Aetna, ATT: American Exp Unit           Note:
        Address.......: Reading, PA   19603
        Phone Number..: (800)641-6444
        Contact.......: Jeff


                          TRANSACTION  FIRST    SECOND  DAYS            INS. PAYM       PROV
   ID        NAME             DATE     BILLED    BILLED UNITS   FEE     EXPECTED  CPT   CODE   COMMENT
 =======  ==============================  ========  ========  ======== ===== ========= ========= =======  == ===============
   90040 BOWER, Julia        Pol#:075-13-9745         Grp#:American Express    Insured:Bower, Julia
                             10/08/90  10/15/90               1    120.00      60.00 90844       KP ck 3115
                             10/15/90  11/02/90               1    120.00      60.00 90844       KP ck 3131
                             10/29/90  11/02/90               1    120.00      60.00 90844       KP ck 3313
                             ----------------------------------------------------------------
                           3 SERVICE(S)       PATIENT TOTAL:   360.00     180.00


 ===================================================================================================================
                           3 SERVICE(S)       INSURANCE TOTAL:  360.00     180.00
 ===================================================================================================================
```

OUTSTANDING INSURANCE REPORT: This report shows unpaid sessions by each insurance company for each patient.

```
                                Psychological Associates
    11/02/90                   INSURANCE EXPIRATIONS REPORT                         Page   1

                  PATIENTS WITH   2 SESSIONS OR     $200.00 FEES (OR LESS) REMAINING
    ===============================================================================================

        Insurance Name: Bl. Cross Bl. Shield              Note:
        Address.......: Jacksonville, FL  32231
        Phone Number..: (904)791-9200
        Contact.......: Jim


    ===============================================================================================
    ID       NAME                     LIFETIME       REMARK      AUTHORIZ. PERIOD     REMARK    AUTH DATE
    ===============================================================================================

      89768 HALL, Arnold              20  used of 999             8  used of 31                 1/01/90
                               $2,010.00 of  $99,999.00      $800.00 of     $750.00  !OVER!
    -----------------------------------------------------------------------------------------------

      89235 JOPLIN, Janet             11  used of 999            11  used of 30                 1/01/90
                               $1,325.00 of  $99,999.00    $1,325.00 of   $1,380.00
    -----------------------------------------------------------------------------------------------

      89373 LEMON, Jeff               16  used of 999            16  used of 52                 1/01/90
                               $1,445.00 of  $99,999.00    $1,445.00 of   $1,250.00  !OVER!
    -----------------------------------------------------------------------------------------------

      89101 MONK, Theodore            12  used of 999            12  used of 99                 1/01/90
                               $1,445.00 of  $99,999.00    $1,445.00 of   $1,350.00  !OVER!
    -----------------------------------------------------------------------------------------------

        Insurance Name: Humana Health Care Plans          Note:
        Address.......: Jacksonville, FL  32245-9080
        Phone Number..: (800)523-0023
        Contact.......: Ron


    ===============================================================================================
    ID       NAME                     LIFETIME       REMARK      AUTHORIZ. PERIOD     REMARK    AUTH DATE
    ===============================================================================================

      81156 BROWN, Jeremy             11  used of 100             5  used of  5                 1/01/90
                               $1,180.00 of  $25,000.00      $580.00 of   $2,500.00
    -----------------------------------------------------------------------------------------------

      84025 REID, Veronica             6  used of 999             6  used of  8                 1/01/90
                                 $720.00 of  $99,999.00      $720.00 of   $9,999.00
    -----------------------------------------------------------------------------------------------

        Insurance Name: Life Of Georgia                   Note:
        Address.......: Atlanta, GA  30348
        Phone Number..: (404)980-5759
        Contact.......: Myrna


    ===============================================================================================
    ID       NAME                     LIFETIME       REMARK      AUTHORIZ. PERIOD     REMARK    AUTH DATE
    ===============================================================================================

      89058 JORDAN, Merrilou          39  used of 999            25  used of 99                 1/01/90
                               $3,910.00 of $999,999.00    $2,500.00 of   $2,100.00  !OVER!
    -----------------------------------------------------------------------------------------------
```

INSURANCE EXPIRATIONS REPORT: This report shows insurance status for each patient by insurance carrier (e.g., status of deductible, sessions authorized, total coverage, remaining coverage, etc.).

REFERENCES

American Medical Association. (1988). *Current Procedural Terminology - CPT-4* (4th ed.). Chicago, IL: Author.

American Psychiatric Association. (1987). *Diagnostic and Statistical Manual of Mental Disorders* (3rd ed. rev.). Washington, DC: Author.

American Psychological Association. (undated-a). *Medicare for Psychologists* (draft handbook). Washington, DC: Author.

American Psychological Association. (undated-b). *Recognition and Reimbursement for Psychological Services*. Washington, DC: Author.

Austad, C. S., DeStefana, L., & Kisch, J. (1988). The health maintenance organization - II. Implications for psychotherapy. *Psychotherapy, 25*(3), 449-462.

Baughman, H. D. (1989). Let's talk about insurance. *Texas Psychologist, 41*(6) 19-20.

Berkman, A. S., Bassos, C. A., & Post, L. (1988). Managed mental health care and independent practice: A challenge to psychology. *Psychotherapy, 25*(3), 415-419.

Bipolar disorder is a physical illness says an Arkansas court. (1988). *Psychotherapy Finances, 15*(5), 8.

Buie, J. (1987, September). Evidence of HMO flaws mounting. *APA Monitor*, p. 45.

Buie, J. (1988, March). New data show HMO dream unfulfilled. *APA Monitor*, p. 18.

Buie, J. (1989a, November). Managed care debate covers pros and cons. *APA Monitor*, p. 21.

Buie, J. (1989b, December). Overzealous Medicaid investigations claimed. *APA Monitor*, p. 21.

California mandates parity for some mental disorders. (1989, October 20). *Psychiatric News*, pp. 1, 15.

Canter, M. B., & Freudenberger, H. J. (1990). Fee scheduling and maintaining. In E. Margenau (Ed.), *The Encyclopedic Handbook of Private Practice* (pp. 217-232). New York: Gardner Press.

Case, M. S. (1990, March 30). Two income families. *How to Get the Most from Your Health Insurances*, pp. 5-6.

CHAMPUS: How poor records pushed a provider into bankruptcy. (1990). *Psychotherapy Finances, 16*(9), 1-4.

Christensen, J. C. (1989, November/December). Play it straight in insurance billing. *Family Therapy News*, p. 9.

Cohen, H. M. (1990). Third party payments. In E. Margenau (Ed.), *The Encyclopedic Handbook of Private Practice* (pp. 233-242). New York: Gardner Press.

Colorado Psychological Association, Insurance Committee. (1983). *Insurance Reimbursement for Psychological Services*. Denver, CO: Author.

Council for the National Register of Health Service Providers in Psychology. (1989, March). Preferred provider organizations - an introduction. *Register Report, 3,* 6.

Council for the National Register of Health Service Providers in Psychology. (1990). Degree v. training: An issue with Hewlett-Packard. *Register Report, 16,* 13, 16.

Court rulings further challenge practice of insurance discrimination of psychiatric disorder. (1989, April 21). *Psychiatric News*, p. 6.

DeLeon, P. H., Vandenbos, G. R., & Kraut, A. G. (1986). Federal recognition of psychology as a profession. In H. Dorken & Associates (Eds.), *Professional Psychology in Transition* (pp. 99-117). San Francisco, CA: Jossey-Bass.

DeSua, J. (1990, March 16). Some advice on how to bill for family consults under Medicare. *Psychiatric News*, p. 14.

Dorken, H. (1986). The expanding role of clinical psychology in the mental health services: The CHAMPUS experience. In H. Dorken & Associates (Eds.), *Professional Psychology in Transition* (pp. 69-98). San Francisco, CA: Jossey-Bass.

Dorken, H., & Wiggins J. G. (1986). Trends in third party reimbursement: How carriers differ. In H. Dorken & Associates (Eds.), *Professional Psychology in Transition* (pp. 44-68). San Francisco, CA: Jossey-Bass.

Dvonch, P. (1990). Vocational rehabilitation. In E. Margenau (Ed.), *The Encyclopedic Handbook of Private Practice* (pp. 333-348). New York: Gardner Press.

Egan, T. (1990, May 3). Oregon lists illnesses by priority to see who gets Medicaid care. *New York Times*, p. 1.

Eliach, J. (1990). How to develop an employee assistance program. In E. Margenau (Ed.), *The Encyclopedic Handbook of Private Practice* (pp. 932-941). New York: Gardner Press.

Ethics Committee of the American Psychological Association. (1988). Trends in ethics cases, common pitfalls and published resources. *American Psychologist, 43*(7) 564-570.

Ewing, C. P. (1990). Legal issues in terminating treatment. In E. Margenau (Ed.), *The Encyclopedic Handbook of Private Practice* (pp. 720-726). New York: Gardner Press.

Facing the challenge of alternative health care systems. (1986). *Psychotherapy Finances, 13*(12) [Special issue].

Feldman, S. L. (1985). *Psychology and HMOs* (Report). Washington, DC: American Psychological Association, Division 38.

Frank, R. G. (1982). "Freedom of choice" laws: Empirical evidence of their contribution to competition in mental health care delivery. *Health Policy Quarterly, 2*(2) 79-97.

Frankel, A. S. (1990). Health care delivery by organized providers. In E. Margenau (Ed.), *The Encyclopedic Handbook of Private Practice* (pp. 442-449). New York: Gardner Press.

Frisman, L. K., McGuire, T. G., & Rosenbach, M. L. (1985). Costs of mandates for outpatient mental health care in private health insurance. *Archives of General Psychiatry, 42*(June), 558-561.

Goldman, W. (1990, May 4). Managed mental health care needs management itself. *Psychiatric News*, pp. 32, 34.

Harran, W. R., VandeCreek, L., & Knapp, S. (1990). Ethical and legal aspects of clinical supervision. *Professional Psychology: Research and Practice, 21*(1), 37-41.

Herrington, B. S. (1989, November 3). Outpatient managed care "inevitable." *Psychiatric News*, pp. 16-17, 22.

Herrington, B. S. (1990, July 6). Pros, cons of managed care aired in annual meeting debate. *Psychiatric News*, pp. 4, 24.

Hewlett-Packard continues to refuse reimbursement to ED.D psychologists. (1990). *Massachusetts Psychologist, 33*(4).

Hinden, R. A. (1988, September). Managed-care entities could be held liable for UR decisions. *Contract Healthcare*, pp. 26-27.

Hogue, E. (1988a). Abandonment: Three elements home care agencies should avoid. *Home Care Economics, 2*(1), 18-21.

Hogue, E. (1988b). Liability for premature discharge. *Pediatric Nursing, 14*(5), 421-423.

Hotchkiss, S. N. (1987). Newman warns of legal responsibility in managed-care programs. *Ohio Psychologist*, pp. 12-13.

Insurance Board v. Muir, 819 F.2d 408 (3rd Cir. 1987).

Insurance information. (1988). *Georgia Psychologist, 41*(1), 23-24.

Jones, S. E. (1982). How to collect insurance reimbursement. In P. A. Keller & L. G. Ritt (Eds.), *Innovations in Clinical Practice: A Sourcebook* (Vol. 1, pp. 184-193). Sarasota, FL: Professional Resource Exchange.

Kiesler, C. A., & Morton, T. L. (1988). Prospective payment system for inpatient psychiatry. *American Psychologist, 43*(3), 141-150.

Kisch, J., & Austad, C. S. (1988). The health maintenance organization - I. Historical perspective and current status. *Psychotherapy, 25*(3), 441-448.

Knapp, S., & VandeCreek, L. (1990). *Pennsylvania Law and Psychology.* Harrisburg, PA: Pennsylvania Psychological Association.

Kovacs, A. L. (1987a). Insurance billing: The growing risk of lawsuits against psychologists. *Independent Practitioner, 7*(May), 21-24.

Kovacs, A. L. (1987b). Psychology as a "health service" profession. *Psychotherapy Bulletin, 24*(1), 13-16.

Kovacs, A. (1988). The changing face of insurance reimbursement. *Georgia Psychologist, 41*(1), 21-26.

Kovacs, A. L. (1989a). Here comes the iceberg. *Psychotherapy Bulletin, 24*(1), 11-14.

Kovacs, A. (1989b). Using ICD-9-CM and CPT-4. *Independent Practitioner, 9*(3), 20.

Koyanagi, C. (1988). *Operation Help: A Mental Health Advocate's Guide to Medicaid.* Alexandria, VA: National Mental Health Association.

Landers, S. (1990, April). HMO MDs overlook depression. *APA Monitor*, pp. 16-17.

Lane, R. C., & Hull, J. W. (1990). The role of fees in psychotherapy and psychoanalysis. In E. Margenau (Ed.), *The Encyclopedic Handbook of Private Practice* (pp. 260-272). New York: Gardner Press.

Langs, R. (1976). *The Bipersonal Field.* New York: Jason Aronson.

Laws of Pennsylvania. (1990). Act 1990-81.

Legal briefing: Why Blue Shield sent a therapist to jail. (1987). *Psychotherapy Finances, 14*(3), 1-2.

Legal issues: Could you be brought up on criminal charges. (1989). *Psychotherapy Finances, 16*(2), 1-3.

Legislation: The slowdown in mandated mental health coverage. (1989). *Psychotherapy Finances, 16*(5), 5.

Managed care court decisions reveal disturbing pattern. (1989, December 1). *Psychiatric News*, pp. 10, 20.

Managed care: Getting along with the new breed of telephone reviewers. (1989). *Psychotherapy Finances, 16*(4), 1-3.

Managed care: Taking a look at how the other side lives. (1990). *Psychotherapy Finances, 16*(9), 4-5.

Managed care: The growing standardization of mental health care. (1989). *Psychotherapy Finances, 16*(5), 1-2.

Margenau, E. (Ed.). (1990). *The Encyclopedic Handbook of Private Practice*. New York: Gardner Press.

Maryland Psychological Association. (1990). *Business Aspects of Psychological Practice: Reimbursement and Insurance Issues*. Columbia, MD: Author.

McGuire T. G. (1981). *Financing Psychotherapy: Costs, Effects and Public Policy*. Cambridge, MA: Ballinger.

McSweeny, J. (1987, December). Don't confuse payment with treatment. *Ohio Psychologist*, p. 12.

Medicare answers to 10 key questions about direct reimbursement. (1990). *Psychotherapy Finances, 16*(10), 1-7.

Medicare: What psychologists and social workers can expect now. (1990). *Psychotherapy Finances, 16*(7), 1-2.

Metropolitan Life Insurance Company v. Commonwealth of Massachusetts, 105 S. Ct. 2380 (1985).

Moran, M. (1990, May 4). Physicians fight Medicaid fraud prosecutions. *Psychiatric News*, pp. 1, 44.

More to change coverage for federal workers has good, bad news for mental health. (1990, Fall). *Practitioner Focus*, p. 5.

Must you help claims people do their jobs. (1989). *Psychotherapy Finances, 16*(3), 7.

Nagle, G. S. (1989, January). Guidelines for submitting insurance claims: Be honest. *Florida Psychologist*, pp. 9-10.

National health plans: What are the chances now. (1979, June). *Psychotherapy Finances*, Section 2.

Nationwide Mutual Insurance Company. (1987, February). Outpatient psychiatric services limitation - "incident to" services. *Medicare Newsletter*, pp. 1-2.

New Medicare fee schedule gets congressional approval. (1989, December 15). *Psychiatric News*, pp. 2, 12-13.

North Carolina Psychological Association Insurance Committee. (1989). *Third Party Reimbursement: An Insurance Manual*. Raleigh, NC: Author.

Office of Civilian and Medical Program of the Uniformed Services. (1988). *CHAMPUS Provider Handbook*. Aurora, CO: Author.

Office of Civilian and Medical Program of the Uniformed Services. (1989, April). *CHAMPUS Mental Health Manual*. Aurora, CO: Author.

Pennsylvania Blue Shield. (1988). *PTM 1988*. Camp Hill, PA: Author.

Pennsylvania Blue Shield. (1989a). *Blue Shield Reference Guide*. Camp Hill, PA: Author.

Pennsylvania Blue Shield. (1989b, Spring). *PRN*. Camp Hill, PA: Author.

Pennsylvania Blue Shield. (1990, April). *Medicare Report*. Camp Hill, PA: Author.

Pennsylvania Blue Shield. (1990-1991, Winter). *Medicare Report*. Camp Hill, PA: Author.

Peres, K. E. (Ed.). (1986) *An Insurance Field Manual for the Psychologist*. Tallahassee, FL: Florida Psychological Association.

Pope, K. (1990). A Practitioner's guide to confidentiality and privilege: 20 legal, ethical and clinical pitfalls. *The Independent Practitioner, 10*(2), 40-45.

Practice building: How to sell EAP programs to small business. (1986). *Psychotherapy Finances, 13*(3), 1-5.

Practice Building: Keeping up with preferred provider organizations - Part 1. (1988). *Psychotherapy Finances, 15*(5), 8.

Practice issues: Answers to basics questions on mental health PPOs. (1989). *Psychotherapy Finances, 16*(5), 3-4.

Practice issues: Ohio psychologists are battling General Motors. (1986). *Psychotherapy Finances, 13*(1), 3.

Practice issues: Social workers now have 16 freedom-of-choice laws. (1987). *Psychotherapy Finances, 14*(4), 4.

Professional issues: GM lowers the boom on psychologists. (1985). *Psychotherapy Finances, 12*(5), 1-2.

Psychotherapy Finances, Herbert E. Klein, Publisher, 422 Lafayette Avenue, Hawthorne, NJ 07506. Telephone: 1-201-427-3366.

Reimbursement: A simple coding system to protect confidentiality. (1985). *Psychotherapy Finances, 12*(2), 1-3.

Reimbursement: Freedom-of-choice continues to spread. (1986). *Psychotherapy Finances, 13*(9), 8.

Reimbursement: Getting paid when a patient's company is self-insured. (1987). *Psychotherapy Finances, 14*(5), 1-2.

Reimbursement: How to handle special situations. (1980). *Psychotherapy Finances, 7*(9), Section 1, 1-3, 7.

Reimbursement: Is private practice threatened by national health insurance. (1979, September). *Psychotherapy Finances*, Section Two.

Reimbursement: Making the most of freedom-of-choice laws. (1985). *Psychotherapy Finances, 12*(8), 6-7.

Rofsky, C. (1989, May 1). Accepting assignment/waiving copayments. *California Psychologist*, p. 6.

Scheidemandel, P. (1989). *The Coverage Catalog* (2nd ed.). Washington, DC: American Psychiatric Press.

Seniors like new law; some doctors don't. (1990, July 11). *Reading (PA) Eagle*, p. 1.

Shulman, M. E. (1988). Cost containment in clinical psychology: Critique of Biodyne and the HMOs. *Professional Psychology: Research and Practice, 19*(3), 298-307.

Small, R. (1987a). Third party payments. *Pennsylvania Psychologist, 46*(1), 7-8.

Small, R. (1987b). Medicare. *Pennsylvania Psychologist, 46*(3), 8.

Small, R. (1987c). Private insurance carriers. *Pennsylvania Psychologist, 46*(6), 6.

Small, R. (1988). Inpatient insurance coverage. *Pennsylvania Psychologist, 47*(1), 6.

Small, R. (1989). Managed care. *Pennsylvania Psychologist, 48*(11), 12-13.

Stimel, C. (1989, November). From the insurance chair. *Florida Psychologist*, p. 5.

Stromberg, C. D., Haggarty, D. J., Leibenluft, R. F., McMillian, M. H., Mishkin, B., Rubin, B. L., & Trilling, H. R. (1988). *The Psychologist's Legal Handbook*. Washington, DC: The Council for the National Register of Health Service Providers in Psychology.

Suit filed in reimbursement discrimination. (1990, February 2). *Psychiatric News*, pp. 1, 15.

Survey of Medicare carriers underscores inadequacy of CPT codes. (1989, November 3). *Psychiatric News*, p. 4.

Tennessee Psychological Association. (1988, November). *General Guidelines for Providers of Psychological Services in Tennessee*. Nashville, TN: Author.

U.S. Department of Health & Human Services Health Care Financing Administration. (1990, August). *Medicare Carrier Manual. Part 3. Claims Process*, pp. 2-86.3 to 2-86.4.

U.S. Department of Labor. (1990). *Health Benefits Under the Consolidated Omnibus Budget Reconciliation Act (COBRA)*. (Pamphlet available from U.S. Department of Labor, Pension and Welfare Benefits Administration, Division of Technical Assistance and Inquiries, 200 Constitution Avenue, N.W. (Room N-5658), Washington, DC 20210.)

Utilization management somewhat effective in controlling inpatient costs, says report. (1989, December 15). *Psychiatric News*, pp. 8, 11.

Vizza, J. (1987). Psychologist participation in HMOs and PPOs. *Psychotherapy in Private Practice, 5*(3) 9-19.

Whiting, L. (1989). *State Comparisons of Laws Regulating Social Work*. Silver Springs, MD: National Association of Social Workers.

Wiggins, J. G. (1987). Self-insurance or selfish insurance. *Psychotherapy in Private Practice, 5*(2), 89-93.

Wiggins, J. G. (1988a). Encoding insurance forms. *Psychotherapy Bulletin, 28*(2), 20-21.

Wiggins, J. G. (1988b). New Medicare benefits for psychotherapy and medical management. *Psychotherapy Bulletin, 23*(11), 9-10.

Wiggins, J. G. (1988c). Some effects of prospective payment by diagnostic related groups on the independent practice of psychotherapy. *Psychotherapy in Private Practice, 6*(1), 63-70.

Wiggins, J. G. (1989a). Managed care: Implications for the psychologist in independent practice. *Independent Practitioner*, pp. 12-13.

Wiggins, J. G. (1989b). Relative value scales and Medicare update. *Psychotherapy Bulletin, 24*(1), 23-24.

Will companies cut mental health care for dependents for drug treatment. (1989). *Psychotherapy Finances, 16*(5), 8.

Wise, E. A. (1988). Issues in psychotherapy with EAP clients. *Psychotherapy, 25*(3), 415-419.

Wishnoff, R. (1990). Employee assistance programs. In E. Margenau (Ed.), *The Encyclopedic Handbook of Private Practice* (pp. 323-332). New York: Gardner Press.

World Health Organization. (1989). *International Classification of Diseases - Clinical Modification* (9th rev., 3rd ed.). Washington, DC: U.S. Department of Health and Human Services.

Wright, R. H. (1990). National health insurance. In E. Margenau (Ed.), *The Encyclopedic Handbook of Private Practice* (pp. 363-371). New York: Gardner Press.

You could be jailed for billing the way some hospitals do it. (1989). *Psychotherapy Finances, 16*(5), 8.

Youngstrom, N. (1990, November). Psychology gets a win with HCFA regulations. *APA Monitor*, p. 18.

Youngstrom, N. (1991, January). Coverage is improved in new UAW contracts. *APA Monitor*, p. 15.

GLOSSARY

Administrator. A company which handles the paperwork and transfer of funds for the actual insurer (e.g., a self-insured trust) or government program. Same as *intermediary*. (See page 9.)

Assignment (of Benefits). Legal authorization by the insured for the insurance company to reimburse the provider directly. (See page 10.)

Beneficiary. The person (not necessarily the patient) eligible for benefits under the insurance contract. Usually synonymous with the *insured*. (See page 15.)

Benefit Period. Usually a 12-month period, often based on the calendar year or contract year. After this time new deductibles must accumulate before benefits will be paid, and yearly benefit limits that were exceeded are not applicable. (See page 28.)

Capitation. Payment to a provider or group of providers, as a set fee for each enrollee, rather than for services rendered. See *Health Maintenance Organization*. (See page 12.)

Carrier. Insurance company or other organization responsible for administration of third-party claims. Carrier sometimes refers only to true insurers and at other times to all third-party reimbursers. (See page 13.)

Carve-Out Benefits. Alternative to traditional coordination of benefits in which secondary carrier reimburses the insured only for the difference between the coverage provided by the primary carrier and the coverage of the secondary insurer. Same as *Maintenance of Benefits*. (See page 13.)

Civilian Health and Medical Program of the Uniformed Services (CHAMPUS). Health care benefit program for families of active and retired military personnel. (See pages 65-67.)

Claim. A request for payment sent by patient or practitioner to a third-party reimburser. (See Chapter 3.)

COBRA (Consolidated Omnibus Budget Reconciliation Act). Cobra provides options for continued group insurance coverage for a limited period of time to employees who have lost group insurance benefits because of job termination or reduced work hours. (See page 54.)

Collateral Visit. Session with a relative, friend, or employer of a patient that is part of the treatment of the patient. (See page 25.)

Coordination of Benefits. A procedure defined by various laws and contract language that provides for payment by the *primary* and *secondary carrier* and prevents patients from being reimbursed for more than the actual cost of care. (See page 13.)

Co-Payment. A fixed amount or percentage, per service, that is the responsibility of the patient, rather than of the third party. (See pages 18 and 36-37.) See also *waiver of co-payment*.

Covered Services. Services defined by the insurance contract as eligible for reimbursement. (See page 55.)

Crime Victim Program. Usually a state-funded program to pay medical and other expenses caused by the crimes of others. (See page 71.)

Customary Charge. The typical fee charged for a service by providers in a community. Both "typical" and "community" may be defined by the insurer. (See page 11.)

Deductible. A specific amount the insured must pay, usually at the beginning of each benefit year, before insurance reimbursement may begin. The deductible may apply to all medical or just mental health benefits. There may be both individual deductibles (e.g., $250) and a family deductible (e.g., $500) so that if either is met, benefits will begin. (See pages 9-10.)

Diagnosis Related Groups (DRGs). Categories of illnesses for which Medicare pays a hospital a set amount, regardless of the actual days and services provided. Seen as a model for other carriers. In the future, DRGs may be extended to individual practitioners. (See pages 62 and 80.)

Diagnostic and Statistical Manual of Mental Disorders, 3rd ed. rev. (DSM-III-R). An American Psychiatric Association manual that lists terminology and diagnosis codes accepted by most insurance companies. (See pages 20-21.) Also see *International Classification of Diseases, 9th ed. (ICD-9-CM)*.

Direct Recognition Statutes. Also known as *Freedom of Choice Laws*, direct recognition statutes require insurance companies that reimburse for services of psychiatrists to reimburse for the same services if provided by other specific providers (usually psychologists, sometimes social workers, and occasionally other mental health professionals). (See pages 11-12 and 45-46.)

Employee Assistance Plan (EAP). Employer-sponsored plans to provide limited counseling services to employees and their families. (See pages 12 and 69-70.)

ERISA (Employees Retirement Income Security Act). ERISA is a Federal law that protects pension benefits but that also allows companies to avoid complying with state insurance mandates when they set up self-insurance trusts. (See pages 11-12 and 47-48.)

Exclusions. Specific illnesses, treatments, or circumstances that are not subject to reimbursement under an insurance contract. (See page 13.)

Extraterritoriality. An exception to *Freedom of Choice Laws* in some states that allows companies with plans written out of state not to comply with provisions of the law. (See pages 46-47.)

Federal Employees Health Benefits Program (FEHB). Series of group health plans covering federal employees. (See pages 67-68.)

Fee for Service. Traditional form of insurance in which the provider is paid for each service performed, as opposed to *capitation*. (See page 9.)

Forgiveness. Also see *waiver of co-payment*.

Fourth Party. Utilization review company hired by a third party. (See pages 12 and 78.)

Freedom of Choice Laws. See *direct recognition statutes*.

Health Maintenance Organization (HMO). A prepaid managed health plan that rewards practitioners for providing as few services as necessary, usually through *capitation*. In principle, HMOs should cut costs by encouraging disease prevention and avoiding unnecessary and expensive procedures. HMOs now take many forms and often are hybrids of *Preferred Provider Organizations* and HMOs. They may use professionals who are their employees or who are in independent practice. Patients must see HMO providers in order to receive any reimbursement. (See pages 12 and 74-75.)

Health Care Financing Administration (HCFA). Government agency that sets regulations for Medicare and other federal programs. (See pages 59-60.)

HCFA-1500. The insurance claim form developed by HCFA. Required for Medicare and accepted by most insurance companies. (See Figure 1, page 16.)

"Incident To" Services. Medicare services provided by a supervisee that are reimbursable. (See pages 38-40.)

Independent Practice Association (IPA). An *HMO* model using practitioners who are not employees of the HMO. (See page 74.)

Individual Provider Profile. An insurance company's record of the *usual* fees charged by a provider over a period of time. (See page 11.)

Insurance. A system of protection against loss in which a number of individuals agree to premiums periodically for a guarantee that they will be compensated under certain conditions for certain losses. (See pages 7-8.)

Insured. See *beneficiary*.

Insurer. The company actually taking the financial risk by promising to pay claims for specified treatments. Insurance companies may serve as insurers or *administrators*. (See pages 7-8.)

International Classification of Diseases, 9th ed. (ICD-9-CM). Mental health portion of international diagnostic listings compiled by the World Health Organization. Most insurance companies accept *ICD-9-CM* listings, which closely parallel those of *DSM-III-R*. (See page 20.)

Intermediary. See *administrator*.

Maintenance of Benefits. Same as *carve-out benefits*.

Managed Care. Attempting to control costs of health care through controls in advance of or during the course of health care. (See page 12 and Chapter 9.)

Major Medical. An adjunct to basic hospitalization and medical services policies that usually adds hospital days, amounts for medical services, and additional services. Outpatient mental health is often covered under major medical provisions. (See page 9.)

Maximums. Limits on the amount of reimbursement per session, per year, or per lifetime. (See page 10.)

Medicaid. Also known as *medical assistance*. A combined federal and state program to provide health services for low-income individuals. (See pages 63-65.)

Medical Assistance. See *Medicaid*.

Medically Necessary. A provision in most health insurance policies that allows the insurer to reimburse only for those treatments that the company deems to be required. (See page 55.)

Medicare. A federal program to provide health services to individuals 65 and older and those with severe disabilities. Part A covers hospital expenses, and Part B covers practitioner fees. (See pages 59-63.)

Medigap. Medicare supplement policies that reimburse the patient for co-payments and deductibles on treatments accepted by Medicare. (See page 61.)

Participating Provider. A practitioner who agrees to see patients enrolled in a program, usually agreeing to accept the insurance company's set reimbursement and usually receiving payment directly from the insurance company. (See page 52.)

Preexisting Condition. An illness that existed before a patient first enlisted in an insurance program. Companies frequently will not pay for preexisting conditions for at least 1 year. (See page 13.)

Preferred Provider Organization (PPO). A managed-care structure with some resemblance to *HMOs* in which participating providers agree to see patients at a lower cost. Patients receive a financial incentive (lower co-payments) for seeing participating providers. (See pages 12 and 75-76.)

Prevailing Charge. Another term for *customary charge*.

Primary Carrier. If a patient is covered by two different policies, the primary carrier has first responsibility for payment. (See page 13.)

Provider. The individual or corporation providing the health service. (See page 25.)

Reasonable Charge. The amount deemed "reasonable" by the insurance company for a particular service. This may be the lower of *usual* and *customary* or an arbitrary figure. To avoid challenges, insurance companies may further limit reimbursement by such statements as "payment will be made for reasonable charges, not to exceed $40 per visit." (See page 11.)

Relative Value Scales. Listings of health care procedures that evaluate their worth compared to each other. (See page 80.)

Secondary Carrier. The insurance company responsible for only that portion left after the *primary carrier* has fulfilled its obligation. This payment may be through *coordination of benefits* or *carve-out benefits*. (See page 13.)

Self-Insured Company. A company that underwrites its own insurance and pays benefits (through an insurance trust) for its employees. These corporations may use insurance companies to administer the plan and may even have insurance for their own catastrophic losses. These plans are usually not subject to state insurance laws but are governed through the federal *ERISA*. (See pages 11-12, 47-48, and 56-57.)

Stop-Loss Limit. A monetary limit above which an insurance plan that was paying a proportion of costs (often 80%) will reimburse subsequent expenses at 100%. Stop-loss limits protect the insured against high co-payments. Mental health benefits are often not afforded stop-loss limits. (See page 10.)

Superbill. A detailed receipt which can also serve as an insurance claim. (See pages 25, 27, and 92.)

Third Party. Any individual or company (e.g., insurance company, employer, parent, friend) who pays part or all of one's health care fees. (See page 7.)

Unique Physician Identification Number (UPIN). An identification number issued by Medicare. Providers are required to identify their own UPIN as well as those of referring providers on all claims. (See p. 63.)

Usual Charge. The most common charge made by a particular practitioner for a particular service over a period of time. (See page 11.)

Usual, Customary, and Reasonable (UCR). A system in which the insurance company pays the lower of the *usual, customary* (prevailing), or *reasonable* charge. (See pages 10-11.)

Utilization Review. A procedure in managed care that usually involves pre-authorizing services, either before treatment begins or after a set number of sessions. (See pages 12 and 77-78.)

Vocational Rehabilitation. Usually a state-funded program designed to help people who have a disability which is a handicap to full and productive employment. (See page 70.)

Waiver of Co-Payment. Charging the insurance company the full fee but not requiring the patient to pay his or her share. (See pages 18 and 36-37). Also known as *forgiveness.*

Workers' Compensation. A program required by all states but administered privately to reimburse employees for illnesses and conditions caused through their employment. (See page 70.)

NOTES

NOTES

Some Of The Other Titles Available
From Professional Resource Exchange, Inc.

Innovations in Clinical Practice: A Source Book - **10 Volumes**
    Hardbound edition (Vols. 3-10 only) per volume.. $54.20
    Looseleaf binder edition (Vols. 1-10) per volume.. $59.20
Cognitive Therapy with Couples... $17.70
Who Speaks for the Children?
    The Handbook of Individual and Class Child Advocacy.. $43.70
Post-Traumatic Stress Disorder: Assessment, Differential Diagnosis, and Forensic Evaluation.. $27.70
Clinical Evaluations of School-Aged Children: A Structured Approach to the Diagnosis of
    Child and Adolescent Mental Disorders.. $22.70
Stress Management Training: A Group Leader's Guide.. $14.70
Stress Management Workbook for Law Enforcement Officers... $ 8.70
Fifty Ways to Avoid Malpractice: A Guidebook for Mental Health Professionals........................ $17.70
Keeping Up the Good Work: A Practitioner's Guide to Mental Health Ethics.............................. $16.70
Think Straight! Feel Great! 21 Guides to Emotional Self-Control.. $14.70
Computer-Assisted Psychological Evaluations: How to Create Testing Programs in BASIC....... $22.70

Titles In Our Practitioner's Resource Series

Assessment and Treatment of Multiple Personality and Dissociative Disorders
Clinical Guidelines for Involuntary Outpatient Treatment
Cognitive Therapy for Personality Disorders: A Schema-Focused Approach
Dealing with Anger Problems: Rational-Emotive Therapeutic Interventions
Diagnosis and Treatment Selection for Anxiety Disorders
Neuropsychological Evaluation of Head Injury
Outpatient Treatment of Child Molesters
Pre-Employment Screening for Psychopathology: A Guide to Professional Practice
Tarasoff and Beyond: Legal and Clinical Considerations in the Treatment of Life-Endangering Patients
What Every Therapist Should Know about AIDS
      (All books in this series are $11.70 each)

To Order

For mail orders, write:
Professional Resource Exchange, Inc.
(Professional Resource Press)
P.O. Box 15560
Sarasota, FL 34277-1560

For fastest service
(Visa/MasterCard/American Express/Discover
or purchase orders only),
CALL 1-813-366-7913
or
FAX 1-813-366-7971

All prices include shipping charges. Foreign orders call or write for shipping information.
All orders from individuals and private institutions must be prepaid in full.
Florida residents add 7%. Prices and availability subject to change without notice.

Please send me:

_____ Copies of *Maximizing Third-Party Reimbursement in Your Mental Health Practice*

List price: $32.70 each (includes shipping)

Canadian and Foreign orders: $33.95 each (includes shipping). *All orders from individuals and private institutions must be prepaid in full.* Florida residents add 7% sales tax. Prices and availability subject to change without notice.

For fastest service
(purchase and credit card orders only)
Call TOLL FREE 1-800-443-3364
Weekdays 9:00 - 5:00 Eastern Time
or
FAX 1-813-366-7971
24 hours a day

Check or money order enclosed (US funds only) $_____

Charge my _____ Visa   _____ MasterCard
           _____ American Express _____ Discover

Card #_____

Exp. Date _____ Daytime Phone # (_____) _____

Signature_____

_____ Order enclosed (ship to name and address below).
_____ Please add my name to your mailing list and send me your latest catalog. (If you ordered this copy from Professional Resource Exchange, Inc. [Professional Resource Press], your name is already on our Preferred-Customer Mailing List.)

Name_____

Address_____

Address_____

City/State/Zip_____

I am a _____ psychologist; _____ clinical social worker; _____ marriage and family therapist; _____ mental health counselor; _____ school psychologist; _____ psychiatrist; _____ other: _____

For mail orders, write:
Professional Resource Exchange, Inc.
(Professional Resource Press)
PO Box 15560
Sarasota, FL 34277-1560

BUSINESS REPLY MAIL
FIRST-CLASS MAIL PERMIT NO. 3084 FT. LAUDERDALE, FL

POSTAGE WILL BE PAID BY ADDRESSEE

Synergistic Office Solutions, Inc.
4801 S. University Drive, Suite 305
Davie, FL 33328-3826

NO POSTAGE
NECESSARY
IF MAILED
IN THE
UNITED STATES

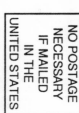

BUSINESS REPLY MAIL
FIRST-CLASS MAIL PERMIT NO 445 SARASOTA FL

POSTAGE WILL BE PAID BY ADDRESSEE

PROFESSIONAL RESOURCE PRESS
PO BOX 15560
SARASOTA FL 34277-9900

NO POSTAGE
NECESSARY
IF MAILED
IN THE
UNITED STATES